Inner Healing

Principles and Universal Laws of Success, Volume 1

Ylich Tarazona

Published by Ylich Eduard Tarazona Gil, 2023.

INNER HEALING

First edition. July 15, 2023.

Copyright © 2023 Ylich Tarazona.

ISBN: 979-8223600299

Written by Ylich Tarazona.

Table of Contents

Dedication

DEDICATION

For you, brave traveler on the path of self-discovery and inner healing. This book is a beacon in the darkness, a guide for those seeking freedom from the invisible chains that bind them. It is a testament to struggle, resistance and victory over self-sabotage, and a reminder that you are not alone in this battle.

In its pages, you will find not only words, but also a reflection of yourself: your fears, your hopes, your dreams. Each chapter, each exercise, each technique has been carefully designed with you, your journey, your transformation in mind.

This book is a tribute to your inner warrior, to that part of you that, despite adversity, keeps fighting, keeps believing, keeps moving forward. It is an invitation to take control of your life, to master your emotions and thoughts, and to walk with determination towards healing and fulfillment.

May these pages serve as a constant reminder of your strength and resilience. May they inspire you to break the chains that bind you and free yourself from self-sabotage. May they help you strengthen your inner warrior and discover the power that resides within you.

This book is for you, with all my love and respect. May it accompany you on your journey, may it bring you comfort in times of doubt, may it inspire you to move forward, always forward, towards the life you deserve and that is waiting for you.

With all my love and respect, your great friend **YLICH TARAZONA**.

Inner Healing

*"**Break Chains and Free Yourself from Inner Self Sabotage.**"*
Learn to Strengthen Your Inner Warrior and Master Your Emotions and Thoughts.

This book is a transformative guide that invites you to embark on a journey of self-discovery and healing. Through its pages, you will learn how to free yourself from emotional self-sabotage, deprogram self-destructive habits and strengthen your inner self.

In this special edition, concepts of Biodescodification and Bioneuroemotion as alternative healing therapies are presented. You will learn to interpret the symbolic meaning of diseases and to balance your energetic points through emotional liberation techniques.

In addition, this book will teach you how to:

- *Understand and take control of your internal battles, allegorically represented by two wolves: one white and one black.*
- *Discover the importance of living in the present and enjoying the journey towards your goals, rather than focusing solely on the destination.*
- *Learn to clean the "garbage" from your mind, freeing yourself from limiting thoughts and emotions.*
- *Admittedly, you are not always in full control of what happens, but you can choose how to react and what actions to take.*
- *Understand that true happiness and meaning in life come from serving others.*

This book is more than just a self-help guide; it is an invitation to take control of your life and awaken the peaceful warrior within you. This book will be your companion on your path to liberation from emotional self-sabotage. Get ready to transform your life with "**Inner Healing**"!

Series: Universal Principles and Laws of Success
First Edition, Volume 2 of 9.
YLICH TARAZONA
Writer and Lecturer

AUTHOR'S RIGHT

This work "**Inner Healing: Break Chains and Free Yourself from Inner Self Sabotage.** *Learn to Strengthen Your Inner Warrior and Master Your Emotions and Thoughts*" is the intellectual property of YLICH TARAZONA.

DEDICATION

For you, brave traveler on the path of self-discovery and inner healing. This book is a beacon in the darkness, a guide for those seeking freedom from the invisible chains that bind them. It is a testament to struggle, resistance and victory over self-sabotage, and a reminder that you are not alone in this battle.

In its pages, you will find not only words, but also a reflection of yourself: your fears, your hopes, your dreams. Each chapter, each exercise, each technique has been carefully designed with you, your journey, your transformation in mind.

This book is a tribute to your inner warrior, to that part of you that, despite adversity, keeps fighting, keeps believing, keeps moving forward. It is an invitation to take control of your life, to master your emotions and thoughts, and to walk with determination towards healing and fulfillment.

May these pages serve as a constant reminder of your strength and resilience. May they inspire you to break the chains that bind you and free yourself from self-sabotage. May they help you strengthen your inner warrior and discover the power that resides within you.

This book is for you, with all my love and respect. May it accompany you on your journey, may it bring you comfort in times of doubt, may it inspire you to move forward, always forward, towards the life you deserve and that is waiting for you.

With all my love and respect, your great friend **YLICH TARAZONA**.

EPIGRAPHS

"**Awaken your inner warrior, free yourself from emotional self-sabotage and take charge of your destiny.**"

"In the battle of life, we are our own warriors. Every thought, every emotion, every action, is a step on the battlefield. But remember, the true warrior is not the one who always wins, but the one who continues to fight despite defeats. This book is a tribute to the warrior in all of us. To the one who, despite adversity, gets up, heals himself and keeps going. Because in the end, the greatest victory is the one achieved over oneself." **YLICH TARAZONA.**

INTRODUCTION

The book "**Inner Healing: Break Chains and Free Yourself from Inner Self Sabotage**" is a profound and transformative guide that takes you on a journey of self-discovery and personal growth. The author, with his unique and compassionate approach, guides you through a healing process that helps you break the chains of your self-imposed limitations and free yourself from self-sabotage.

The book is divided into several sections, each focusing on a different aspect of inner healing. From understanding your emotions and thoughts, to strengthening your inner warrior, the book provides you with the tools and techniques necessary to take control of your life and reach your full potential.

The author uses a combination of theory and practice, providing exercises, techniques, and methodologies that you can apply in your daily life. In addition, the book also incorporates elements of alternative therapies, providing a holistic perspective on healing and personal growth.

"In the depths of our being, we all carry chains. Chains of fear, of doubt, of insecurity. Chains that limit us, that keep us trapped in patterns of thought and behavior that prevent us from reaching our true potential. But what if you could break those chains? What if you could free yourself from self-sabotage and embrace your true self?

Welcome to "**Inner Healing: Break Chains and Free Yourself from Inner Self Sabotage**". This is not just a book; it is a journey. A journey of self-discovery and personal growth. A journey that will take you to the depths of your being and help you unravel the mysteries of your mind and emotions.

Throughout this journey, you will learn to strengthen your inner warrior, master your emotions and thoughts, and free yourself from the chains that have kept you bound. With practical exercises, proven techniques and a holistic perspective on healing, this book will provide you with the tools you need to transform your life.

So, open your mind, open your heart, and get ready to embark on the most important journey of all: the journey to your inner healing."

In your hands you hold a book that is not just a book, it is a key. A key that opens the door to a journey of self-discovery and inner healing. "**Inner**

Healing: Break Chains and Break Free from Inner Self Sabotage" is a guide for those seeking to break free from the invisible chains that keep them bound to destructive patterns of thought and behavior.

This book is a call to awaken the inner warrior in all of us. A warrior that is strong, resilient, and capable of facing and overcoming any challenge that life may present. But before you can awaken this warrior, you must face yourself, your fears, your insecurities, your emotions, and thoughts.

Through a series of exercises, techniques and methodologies, this book will guide you on a journey of self-discovery and self-knowledge. It will help you understand and accept your emotions, change your thought patterns, and free yourself from the chains of self-sabotage.

But this book is not only a guide, but it is also a mirror. A mirror that will show you what you really are, not what you think you are, not what others think you are, but what you really are. And once you see yourself as you are, you will be able to change, to grow, to heal.

So, I invite you to open this book, open your mind and heart, and embark on this journey of inner healing. It will not be an easy journey, but I promise you it will be a journey worth taking. Because at the end of the road, you will find not only healing, but also freedom. The freedom to be yourself, to live your life your way, to be the master of your emotions and thoughts.

PREFACE BY THE AUTHOR

Dear reader:

In the pages that follow, I invite you to embark on a journey of self-discovery and transformation. This book, **"Inner Healing: Break Chains and Free Yourself from Inner Self Sabotage"**, is more than just words on paper. It is a guide, a map that will take you through the recesses of your mind and emotions, helping you to strengthen your inner warrior and master your thoughts and emotions.

We all carry chains, some visible, some not. These chains are our fears, our doubts, our self-sabotage patterns that prevent us from reaching our true potential. This book will teach you how to break these chains, how to free yourself from self-imposed limitations and how to heal from within.

Through a series of exercises, techniques, and methodologies, you will learn to face and overcome your fears, change your thought patterns, and cultivate a growth mindset and self-affirmation. This book will provide you with the tools you need to initiate deep and lasting change in your life.

But this journey is not easy. It requires courage, determination, and an unwavering will to change. But I promise you, the journey is worth it. Because at the end of the road, you will find a stronger, more resilient, and more at peace with yourself.

So, I invite you to open your mind and heart to the possibilities this book has to offer. I invite you to break your chains, to free yourself from self-sabotage and embark on the journey of inner healing. Because at the end of the day, the only person who can heal you is yourself.

Are you ready to break the chains and free yourself from self-sabotage? Are you ready to awaken your inner warrior and master your emotions and thoughts? If your answer is yes, then this book is for you. So, without further ado let's get started.

CHAPTER I: BECOMING AWARE OF OUR INNER WARRIOR

Part One: Understanding Our Inner Battles

Hello, how are you? A big greeting. Once again, we meet here through this wonderful medium that I have to share with you great and extraordinary teachings.

In this opportunity, I am going to share with you a topic that will forever challenge the way we have healed ourselves. We will do this by taking control of our actions, emotions, and thoughts.

In this special edition of this book, you will learn how to heal yourself and free yourself from emotional self-sabotage. Which are nothing more than internal battles that are fought inside your mind at every moment.

Here, through this book that I have prepared, I will share with you in an allegorical way certain principles that govern internal self-sabotage and emotional healing. So that through metaphorical representations in conjunction with more specific topics we can break down step by step the main idea of this great new challenge.

To get into the subject of this first part of the book, which I called: Becoming aware of our inner warrior and understanding our inner battles, I am going to do it through one of the most powerful methodologies of NLP, Ericksonian hypnosis and ontological coaching. I am going to do it through one of the most powerful methodologies of NLP, Ericksonian hypnosis and ontological coaching. Which is metaphoric language.

In this opportunity I am going to start sharing with you an old Sioux legend, which I learned some years ago. And even today, its profound message is still as valid as the first time I heard it.

It is an ancient story of indigenous wisdom that reveals great truths about our inner battles. Battles that take place inside our mind. This story allows us to understand in an allegorical way the importance of taking control of our inner warrior in the struggle to free ourselves from our inner emotional self-sabotage.

-The Legend of the 2 Wolves".

*An ancient legend tells that long ago there was an old chieftain of a Sioux tribe, who was having a mystical conversation about the mysteries of life. The old chieftain related that: "**A great battle is going on inside our mind; and that it was between 2 powerful rival warriors. One was a white wolf and the other a black wolf**".*

The cacique elder continued with his teaching and said that one of the rivals, the black wolf, personifies evil, fear, anger, envy, pain, rancor, greed, arrogance, guilt, and resentment. As well as the feeling of inferiority, lies, hatred, pride, selfishness, superiority, negative thoughts and all those limiting emotions that besiege us to destroy us if possible.

While, on the other hand, the second warrior or white wolf represented goodness, joy, peace, happiness, love, charity, hope and faith. It also represents serenity, humility, gentleness, generosity, compassion, mercy, friendship, and sincerity. As well as positive thoughts and all those empowered emotions that allow us to develop the maximum of our human potential. Empowering us to take our lives to the next higher level of consciousness in divine harmony with the infinite source called God.

And this same battle, my children, is occurring within each one of you. And it is also happening in the same way within each of all human beings who inhabit this earth.

Once this part of the story was told, the old chieftain fell silent as if to give the tribe enough time to understand the profound and mystical teaching. The children who were also gathered listening to the story thought for a few moments and after a few moments one of the grandchildren curiously asked his grandfather and said: "Grandfather, tell us, which of the two wolves do you think will win?

And the old chieftain, looking his grandchildren in the eyes and making eye contact with all the other members of the tribe, replied: my children, the warrior who will win and the wolf who will win this great battle will be the one who you simply feed the most with your thoughts, feelings, emotions, and actions.

After reading this ancient Sioux legend and reflecting on its mystical indigenous wisdom, we were able to learn that it reveals great truths about our inner battles. Battles that take place inside our mind and represent the two opposing sides of every human being. The good and the bad, as well as the positive and the negative. Understanding this principle of duality between the two contenders, the white wolf, and the black wolf, allows us to glimpse in an allegorical way the importance of taking control of our inner warrior in the struggle to free ourselves from inner emotional self-sabotage.

*** Exercise Number 1: Taking Control of Our Internal Battles.**

In the following lines I invite you to write down the teachings you learned in this story and detail the actions you are going to take to feed your inner warrior or white wolf. And in this way begin to heal your life and take control of your thoughts and emotions.

Remember that everything is in our mind, everything is in our thoughts, feelings, and actions. When we decide to take the first step and courageously face our inner self-sabotage, emotional or black wolf. God, the divine source, universal energy, and destiny will begin to conspire in our favor, providing us with the circumstances, events, and actions we need to win in this great internal battle.

Once we have correctly chosen to feed the white wolf and give courage to the warrior that we all carry within us. Then it is there that our great victory against our true rival, ourselves, will begin.
- Ylich Tarazona.

Part Two: The 10 Teachings of the Pacific Warrior

As we have learned in the previous story, we all battle in our mind and in our consciousness with two great rivals. One of them is allegorically personified by a "**Black Wolf**", bringing a check on negative thoughts, and limiting emotions. While, on the other hand, we have a great inner warrior metaphorically represented by a "**White Wolf**" which refers to positive thoughts and our most empowering emotions. Thoughts and emotions that allow us to heal ourselves and develop our fullest human potential by bringing our faculties to a new, higher level of consciousness.

Something interesting to note is that the only ones who feed both warriors and rivals that exist within us are ourselves. And we do it through our thoughts, feelings, and actions... So, the question we should ask ourselves is: which of the two wolves are we feeding?

While writing this first chapter entitled "**Becoming aware of our inner warrior and understanding our inner battles**" an excellent movie I saw some years ago came to my mind and I like it very much for the teaching it imparts, especially for the message it conveys. I have used the teaching of this movie as an allegory in many of my conferences, both face-to-face and virtual.

It is an extraordinary true-life story of Dan Millman a former martial arts master athlete, coach, and university professor. This story allows us to better understand the ancient Sioux legend of the two wolves and is useful to introduce the main teaching of this book. That is the theme of Healing ourselves and freeing ourselves from internal emotional self-sabotage.

The movie I am referring to is called Peaceful Warrior. The movie is based on the best-selling book of the same name. The movie was a box office hit in 2006 directed by Victor Salva, starring Scott Mechlowicz (Dan Millman) and Nick Nolte (Socrates). The film is a story of transformational change and personal and spiritual overcoming.

The film is about an athlete named Dan Millman who is preparing to participate in the Olympics. This character begins to be egomaniacal of himself, that is to say, presumptuous, vain and selfish. And as in any film with an excellent script, another main character appears, Socrates, who personifies a kind of mentor, philosopher guide and spiritual master who wants to teach a profound truth to the protagonist.

Among the most important teachings of the movie "The Peaceful Warrior" we can mention the following:

1. "Be fully present in this moment here and now. It is the first teaching of "Socrates" to his disciple and possibly one of the most powerful. You only have the present... Sometimes there are people who self-sabotage themselves by thinking about future adversities, causing them anxiety because they focus on what they do not want to happen instead of focusing on what they do want to achieve and what they could conquer if they set their mind to it.

In many other cases they focus their thoughts, emotions, and memories on the past and as a result this produces remorse for not having acted differently than they could have instead of focusing on what they did learn and how those life lessons will help them improve their present with the same experience.

One of the messages of the movie teaches us that in order to win in the battlefield of our thoughts and emotions that is constantly going on inside our mind, what we must do first is to manage to live in the present in the here and now. You would be surprised how much you can heal yourself and how much you can accomplish and how good you can feel if you live in the present every moment preparing for the future.

Remember that each moment is unique, there are never empty moments. The peaceful warrior is the one who knows how to enjoy every moment of his life, the one who can focus on the here and now and make the most of every present moment of his life. When we are able to free ourselves and overcome the influence exerted by the black wolf by focusing our attention on the present, not only will we do everything much better, but we will also feel more comfortable, since the white wolf will enter the scene. And you, are you fully enjoying your present?

2. "The journey brings happiness, not the destination". In other words, "happiness is not in the goal we want to achieve, but happiness is on the way to the goal". Are you happy? This is the first question "Socrates" chooses to ask his new friend. We look for happiness in material achievements, in social, academic, labor recognition, etc. But that is either limited or depends on external factors over which we can do nothing.

Happiness if it is anywhere within each one of us and it is part of the white wolf that we have to learn to make it part of our daily life. If we become obsessed with the destination or the goal, we forget to enjoy the journey or the road to the goal. And in the end the journey is what really brings us happiness because every moment is unique and finally every experience in life is part of what will enrich the destination or goal once we have achieved it. And you, are you enjoying your journey and the road to the goal?

3. "Get the garbage out of your mind". This is another of the great teachings of "Socrates" to his young disciple. The garbage represents the black wolf and all those limiting thoughts and emotions that distract you from what is really important. If we understood the power of our positive thoughts and empowered emotions represented by the white wolf to help us overcome any setbacks and heal our lives. If we became aware of this principle, we would be able to clear the "garbage" of the countless useless thoughts that come and go at high speed through the mind, freeing us from internal emotional self-sabotage and thus live life as it is and not what we pretend it to be. And you, have you already removed the garbage from your mind?

4. "Life is choice and decision. You can choose to be a victim or decide to be a warrior and win your internal or external battles". In our hands is the decision to choose between living in the present as true warriors or white wolves preparing for the future or living in the past as victims of adversities and rivals of ourselves living in the past as the black wolf. From the present you will realize that "there are many things to win" because you are a warrior, and you were born to succeed. But if you live clinging to the past, you will be afraid of losing and you will not have enough courage to win your battles when they arise. And you, have you already decided to choose to be a warrior?

5. "**Avoid spending so much time planning and spend more time acting and making things happen.** The real battles take place inside our mind between that black wolf focused on self-sabotage and your truest self, represented by the white wolf, a deeper warrior focused on balancing thoughts and emotions. We must begin to take action, take action and make things happen. Remember "a true peaceful warrior or white wolf acts, while the ego personified in the black wolf overacts". Being a warrior does not mean being perfect and victorious in every battle or being invulnerable in the face of adversity.

The true warrior is one who recognizes his weaknesses on the mental battlefield or internal emotional self-sabotage and works on them, while at the same time focusing on his strengths and healing his life. A true warrior is the one who learns to live wisely in truth, is fundamentally a simple person, focused on his principles and who acts or takes action when any adverse circumstance appears in life. And you, have you already decided to choose, act, and take action?

6. "**We must accept that one does not always have total control of what happens. The important thing is to do what you are passionate about, without attachment to results".** We must take risks without fear of failure, just act, and make things happen without being attached to a result but focus on actions that will produce better achievements as a consequence. A true warrior or white wolf never gives up on what he is passionate about, because he finds love in everything he does, he simply acts and enjoys the process of taking action and making things happen. And you, do you already know what you love and started doing what you are passionate about?

7. "**Be more than you think and think more than you know.** Knowledge does not equal wisdom. Knowledge is what we know, intelligence is how we apply what we know, and wisdom is living what we know and teach. You are

not your thoughts; you are the one who thinks. That is, you become what you focus on with your thoughts. For this reason, we should choose wisely what to focus our thoughts and emotions on. Not knowing what to believe is already a good start because when we begin to choose what to think, it allows us to reflect and make better decisions about how we act in life. Be wise; don't be satisfied only with the knowledge of what you know. Be smart and learn to apply that knowledge to what you do. As you become wise, you live what you teach. This is the big difference between the black wolf that only reacts to its environment (thought + emotion = result) and the white wolf that responds focused on what it perceives and knows is right (thought + emotion + analysis + action = result). Have you decided to act and take wise action?

8. "Death is not sad. What is sad is that people do not know how to live". Many people are saddened by the death of a close relative because that person ceases to exist on this earth. But few people question how they are living their own lives. Many people go through their existence without thinking about whether they are really alive and awake. One can live a whole life without ever being awake or, in other words, one can survive a whole life without ever really living it. Worst of all, many warriors stop fighting for their dreams and allow their rival, the black wolf, to take control of their lives. As a consequence, such actions are responsible for the extinction of their greatest ally, the white wolf. Have you woken up and are you really living? Which of the two wolves are you feeding?

9. "People are not what they think they are. They only think they are. This is another profound truth that the wise teacher Socrates teaches his good friend. We tend to identify ourselves with our past experiences, current lives, or professions, or with the experiences of the future. For example: past experiences such as "I was a great engineer, an outstanding lawyer, a good student, I was the husband of"; present lives or professions such as "I am a consultant, I am a doctor, I am a politician, I am the father or mother of"; future experiences such as "I will be rich", "I will be recognized", "I will have such and such", "I will take the place of". All this argumentation configures what we call our "ego". But we are not the ego, we are what we are now, and we are in the present. Men and women of great value in the eyes of a supreme being, whether we recognize it or not. Sometimes many people choose an identity that they have assumed to be real and that supposedly gives meaning to their lives. They set those assumptions as something that marks their paths, and they stick to those self-sabotaging beliefs. The worst thing is that they are afraid to give that up. Why else are they that? What are they? Internal self-sabotage is that which is ruled by the black wolf that makes us believe we are superior or inferior to others, creating internal or external conflict and rivalry between ourselves and the people around us. We must keep in mind that we are what we decide to be, and we become what we consider ourselves to be. The most essential thing in this life is to be what we want to be without attachment to material recognition or the flattery of the world. Do you already know who you are and what you want to become?

10. "**What has true meaning in our lives is what we are in the service of others.** In the movie Socrates teaches his friend this great truth when his friend questioned his wisdom as a spiritual guide or teacher because of his work at the service station. Socrates then took the opportunity to teach him that to serve is a privilege. There is no greater purpose than to serve others. No one is more or better or worse than anyone else because of what he or she does. In other words, no one is inferior or superior to another because of what he or she performs. True warriors are those who decide to choose to be what they are passionate about doing and allow the white wolf to guide their lives in favor of service and in love for their fellow man. Later in the film, Socrates teaches his young disciple another great truth when he said, "You will never be better than anyone else, just as you will never be worse than anyone else...it is all a matter of habit." True warriors are those who manage to be the best they can be in comparison to their own achievements and by overcoming their own internal battles with themselves.

In the movie we can learn that humility is a quality that represents true warriors and love as well as service to others is a virtue that symbolizes a true white wolf. That is why we should always be attentive to cultivate and develop those qualities in ourselves. Remember: The one who costs the most to love is the one who needs the most love. Have you already decided to serve others without expecting anything in return? Are you humbling enough to love your neighbor?

* **Points to consider**:

To conclude with the teachings of the film, I will share with you another of the truths that the wise Socrates taught his young disciple so that he could learn to discover for himself the answer to all these questions. One way he did this was by teaching him "The Three Rules of Life":

First: The paradox. Life is a mystery, never waste your valuable time deducing it, just live it to the fullest.

Second: Humor. Never lose your sense and above all the sense of humor in yourself, as this will give you colossal strength in the face of adversity.

Third: Change. Everything transmutes and changes form, there is nothing that lasts in the same state, change is part of life itself.

*** Final words**:

In closing, I am going to invite you to download and watch the movie "The Peaceful Warrior" and learn for yourself the original teachings in it. Since, for the practical purposes of this book, I took only some of the main teachings and adapted them to the main theme which is: healing we and freeing ourselves from inner emotional self-sabotage. Therefore, by only taking part of the teachings, I have left aside many other important teachings contained in this great and wonderful cinematographic work. I hope you liked this compendium I made of "**The 10 Teachings of the Pacific Warrior**" and the fusion I made between the film and the Ancient Sioux Legend of the Two Wolves, the Black and the White. The purpose of having begun my book in this way is to transmit to you in a metaphorical way the profound teaching that I wish to teach you next and that we will analyze in more detail in the following chapters.

*** Exercise Number 2: Becoming aware of our peaceful warrior.**

We will continue with a brief summary of the teachings of the Peaceful Warrior and write about how to apply each of these principles to your own life.

To be fully present in this moment, here and now". This is Socrates' first teaching to his disciple and possibly one of the most powerful. You only have the present... Are you fully enjoying your present?

2.- "The journey brings happiness, not the destination". In other words, "happiness is not in the goal we want to achieve but on the way to the goal". Are you happy? This is the first question Socrates chose for his new friend. We look for happiness in material achievements, in social, academic, labor recognition, etc. But that is limited or depends on external factors that we can do nothing about. Are you enjoying the journey and the road to the goal?

3.- "Get the garbage out of your mind". This is another of Socrates' great teachings to his young disciple. Garbage represents the black wolf and all those limiting thoughts or emotions that distract us from what is really important. Have you already taken the garbage out of your mind?

Life is choice and decision; you can choose to be a victim or decide to be a warrior and win your internal and external battles". In our hands is the decision to choose between living in the present as true warriors or white wolves, preparing for the future, or living in the past as victims of adversities and rivals of ourselves, living in the past as the black wolf. Have you already decided to choose to be a warrior?

Avoid spending so much time planning and invest more time in acting and making things happen" You have to start, act and make things happen. Remember: "A true warrior or white wolf acts, while the ego, personified in the black wolf, overacts". Being a warrior does not mean being perfect and victorious in every battle or being invulnerable in the face of adversity. The true warrior is one who recognizes his weaknesses on the mental battlefield or internal emotional self-sabotage and works on them while focusing on his strengths. Have you already decided to choose to act and take action?

We must accept that we do not always have total control of what happens. The important thing is to do what you are passionate about without attachment to results". A true warrior or white wolf never gives up on what he is passionate about, since he finds love in everything he does. Just take action and enjoy the process of taking action and making things happen. Do you already know what you love and have you started doing what you are passionate about?

7.- "Be more than you think and think more than you know". Knowledge does not equal wisdom. Knowledge is what we know, intelligence is how we apply what we know, while wisdom consists of living what we know and teach. Be wise; don't be satisfied with just the knowledge of what you know. Be smart and learn to apply that knowledge in what you do. As you become wise, you live what you teach. Have you already decided to act and take wise action?

8.- "Death is not sad. What is sad is that people do not know how to live". You can live a whole life without ever being awake or, in other words, you can survive a whole life without ever really living it. Have you woken up and are you really living? Which of the two wolves are you feeding?

People are not what they think they are. They only think they are". This is another profound truth that the wise master Socrates teaches his good friend. We tend to identify ourselves with our past experiences, present lives, or professions, or with the experiences of the future. We must keep in mind that we are what we choose to be, and we become what we think of who we are. The most essential thing in this life is to be what we want to be without attachment to material recognition or the flattery of the world. Do you already know who you are and what you want to become?

10.- "What has true meaning in our lives is what we are in the service of others". In the movie Socrates teaches his friend this great truth when he questioned his wisdom as a spiritual guide or teacher because of his work at the service station. Socrates then took the opportunity to teach him that to serve is a privilege. There is no greater purpose than to serve others. Have you already decided to serve others without expecting anything in return? Are you humbling enough to love your fellow man? I never said it would be easy, but I promise you it won't be impossible either... you just have to be willing to pay the price of success and then enjoy the results for the rest of your life. - Ylich Tarazona.

CHAPTER II: BREAKING FREE FROM INTERNAL EMOTIONAL SELF-SABOTAGE

Part One: Internal Emotional Self-Sabotage.

In this second chapter, I am going to teach you the principles of Biodescodification and Bioneuroemotion, which are useful tools to manage emotions more efficiently. Both Biodescodification and Bioneuroemotion work with emotions such as pain, guilt, fear, revenge, anger, rage, doubt, fear, sadness, remorse, jealousy, attachments, fear of failure and fear of success, among other negative feelings and behaviors.

These stagnant emotions can produce psychosomatic illnesses and internal emotional self-sabotage that prevent us from continually progressing in our journey through life. These limiting emotions in their many variants do not allow you to move forward. Some of them become stronger over time and create distortions and irrational interpretations of life. In many cases they can even produce psychosomatic illnesses.

Before continuing, I want to share with you a brief definition of emotional internal self-sabotage, which is and will be the objective of study in this second chapter of the book. Emotional internal self-sabotage is basically that undesirable mental state in which our thoughts and feelings are determined to prevent us from achieving our dreams and goals. The simplest example is the person who wants to lose weight, but at the first opportunity is tempted by a cupcake. He eats it, postpones his diet, and does not continue with the goal he had set for himself: to lose weight.

Even self-sabotage can come in the form of that little voice or internal self-critical thought that appears when you start doing an activity that you know is important to you. However, despite how valuable that activity may be, you end up putting it off or putting it aside without realizing that you have self-sabotaged yourself with limiting thoughts and emotions such as "I'd better start tomorrow", "this is not for me", "it works for other people, but not for me". In other actions, that same inner voice and negative thoughts speak to you in the third person with ideas such as "you don't know how to do that", "you can't do that", "you were not born with those qualities", "you are not capable of...".

As we could appreciate in the previous examples, the internal emotional self-sabotage can appear in different events or in different ways, causing in most cases illnesses, fear of failure, lack of action and even discouragement, self-depression, or procrastination. It is for this reason that it is important to learn how to heal yourself and free yourself from that internal emotional self-sabotage by releasing those energetic charges, negative thoughts or limiting emotions and drain those psychic blockages that are produced in the subconscious mind.

One of the most recommended ways by experts to begin this process of healing and liberation is to explore what is the cause that originated that internal emotional self-sabotage and try to discover what was the reason that originated that inner voice. What activated that negative thought, limiting emotion or energetic charge that produced that subconscious blockage. Once we have determined what was the reason that produced such internal commotion.

The first step we must take is to acknowledge that emotion and accept it, whether it is anger, fear, guilt, hurt, hate, procrastination, or anxiety. The second step is to reconcile with yourself and give yourself permission to forgive yourself and let go of any attachments that caused the incident. The third and final step is to completely disconnect yourself from that energetic charge, negative thought or limiting emotion that has occurred and close that cycle, letting new energy and positive thoughts flow with a feeling of peace, joy, and happiness along with the determination to completely free yourself from that which produced the internal emotional self-sabotage.

It is important to remember at this point that we all have to some extent a mental battle or internal emotional self-sabotage. To a greater or lesser degree, the vast majority of people must deal with feelings, whether of pain, guilt, fear, fear, revenge, anger, rage, hatred or remorse, as well as dealing with doubt, sadness, jealousy, attachments, fear of failure, fear of success and procrastination among others. Emotions condensed with thoughts, feelings and bad actions that are represented by that big black wolf.

You have to understand that this inner sabotage is the one that opens the door to those limiting negative thoughts, feelings or behaviors, without considering the emotional imbalance that these can cause in the mind, body and spirit of the individual. This internal emotional self-sabotage is the one that makes you hesitate between taking action and focusing on your goals or staying in inaction and postponing the execution of your plans due to lack of purpose. Many other times for fear of the unknown or fear, either of success or failure, producing procrastination which is the habit of postponing your decisions. And this action finally produces a stagnation in your progress or a mental block that is reflected in your attitude, character, and personality, therefore, in your way of proceeding in life.

By learning to heal ourselves and free us from internal emotional self-sabotage we will be able to develop nobler and more virtuous feelings such as forgiveness, repentance, gratitude, service, and love, which is the most powerful quality or force in the universe. In this way, by learning to develop these attributes we will begin to expand our consciousness, amplify our connection with the divine and connect with our inner warrior or white wolf, attracting to our life new realities, situations, people, and events according to our new predominant positive thoughts that are definitely the creators of our history and forgers of our destiny.

Although our inner self-saboteur is associated with negative feelings and limiting emotions or behaviors, not entirely pleasant or enjoyable, its presence should not always be taken as something counterproductive necessarily. Let me explain why... After all, each and every one of us, that is, you and me, has something to learn from our inner battles or emotional self-sabotage.

It is important to remember that many of these negative feelings, thoughts or behaviors are only a reflection of our emotions, as well as the repetition of certain habits or mental, neurobiological conditioning, which are the result of programming and limiting thought patterns. When they appear consecutively and permanently in our way of life, they communicate to us that there is something inadequate that we must improve or correct.

When internal emotional self-sabotage is presented in the form of formed thoughts, either by your beliefs, ideas, experiences, or opinions, we must channel and channel them to our own advantage, learning to listen to that inner voice and recognize what is the reason why it was present. Then it is there where we can begin to work on those emotions, heal, forgive, repent, and free ourselves.

"When you do what you fear most and manage to overcome your fears, you learn to do anything" - **Stephen Richards**.

"You can have anything you want if you are willing to give up the limiting belief that you can't achieve it" - **Dr. Robert Anthony**.

"Only when you learn to conquer yourself do you begin to conquer your outside world" - **Ylich Tarazona**.

*** Necessary steps to stop self-sabotage:**

Awareness: This involves recognizing when, where how and why the self-sabotage occurs, assuming your responsibility at the moment of realizing the reason for its occurrence and taking action to correct the self-limiting situation immediately.

2. **Change management**: Immediately set aside any negative feeling, limiting emotion or critical thought when it appears, channeling and channeling it to your own advantage, learning to listen to that inner voice and recognizing the reason why it was present. Once we become aware of the situation, we reconcile with ourselves, this action gives us the freedom to let go of any attachment that caused the incident.

3. **Keep moving forward**: Disconnect completely from that energetic charge, negative thought or limiting emotion that has occurred, then close that cycle, letting new, more empowered energies flow, creating positive thoughts, and acting decisively and confidently having full assurance that you are in control of the situation.

Part Two: Understanding and Deactivating Internal Emotional Self-Sabotage

Throughout our lives, we have been conditioned by experiences, family and social influences, and our inner thoughts. Often, these factors play a significant role in creating our patterns of emotional self-sabotage. To defuse internal emotional self-sabotage, we must deeply understand these conditioning factors, and work on dismantling the beliefs and thought patterns that lead us to sabotage our own efforts.

First, it is essential to understand that our thought patterns are shaped by our previous experiences and conditioning. When we adopt these beliefs and patterns, they often prevent us from perceiving other ways of thinking and acting. They can limit our ability to recognize and take advantage of opportunities, and instead cause us to fall into patterns of self-sabotage.

For example, if we have been conditioned to believe that we are not worthy of success, we may sabotage our chances of success without even realizing it. This can manifest itself in many ways, such as procrastinating, avoiding taking risks, and even turning down opportunities that could lead to success.

To deactivate internal emotional self-sabotage, we must begin by identifying our limiting beliefs and thought patterns. It is important to pay attention to our thoughts and observe how they influence our actions. By doing this, we will begin to notice the patterns of thought and behavior that lead to self-sabotage.

Once we have identified these beliefs and patterns, we can begin to dismantle them. This can be done through various techniques, such as cognitive-behavioral therapy, meditation, yoga, or even just talking to someone we trust about our thoughts and feelings.

It is essential to remember that this process of deactivating internal emotional self-sabotage does not happen overnight. It is a journey that requires commitment, patience, and self-compassion. There is nothing wrong with asking for help when we need it, and sometimes the guidance of a professional can be invaluable in this journey.

Last but not least, we must remember that we are all human and we all make mistakes. Self-sabotage is not a reflection of our value as people, but simply a behavioral pattern that we can change. By learning to deactivate internal emotional self-sabotage, we will not only be helping ourselves to achieve our goals, but we will also be improving our quality of life.

The path to freedom from inner emotional self-sabotage can be challenging, but it can also be incredibly rewarding. With each small step we take on this journey, we are getting closer and closer to living a freer, fuller, more authentic life. And that, dear reader, is a gift we all deserve.

*** Practical tools for emotional liberation.**

After addressing in depth, the importance of freeing ourselves from internal emotional self-sabotage and the many reasons why we should embark on this journey of self-discovery and healing, it is essential to provide some practical and effective strategies to begin navigating this process.

Here are some of the tools most commonly used by experts and people who have successfully overcome emotional self-sabotage. Each of these methods has the potential to help you identify, dismantle, and ultimately overcome the limiting patterns that are holding you back.

Self-observation: Learning to observe yourself is an invaluable skill in the process of freeing yourself from emotional self-sabotage. By paying attention to your thoughts, emotions, and behaviors, you will be able to identify patterns that lead to self-sabotage. This mindful self-observation will allow you to interrupt these patterns and begin to change them into healthier, more beneficial habits.

Meditation: Meditation can be a very useful tool to calm your mind and cultivate greater awareness of your thoughts and emotions. It will allow you to disidentify from destructive patterns and achieve a more balanced and serene state of mind.

3. **Breathing Techniques**: Mindful breathing can help you calm your nervous system, reduce stress, and facilitate greater mental clarity. This can be especially helpful in times of high stress when self-sabotaging patterns tend to be strongest.

4. **Reflective Writing**: Keep a journal where you can write down your thoughts and emotions. This process of self-reflection can help you identify and better understand your self-sabotaging patterns. In addition, writing can be therapeutic, helping you release negative emotions and thoughts.

5. **Therapy or Coaching**: Working with a trained professional can be extremely beneficial in the process of freeing yourself from emotional self-sabotage. They can provide you with a safe space to explore your emotions and thoughts, and offer tools and strategies tailored to your specific needs.

6. **Positive Affirmations**: Positive affirmations are statements you make to reprogram your thoughts. By repeating these statements on a regular basis, you can begin to change your negative and limiting beliefs into more positive and powerful thoughts.

Remember, these tools are not a magic cure, but they are an excellent starting point on your path to freedom from inner emotional self-sabotage. The process of healing and change is a journey, it takes time, patience, and a willingness to face yourself in ways that may be uncomfortable or challenging. But you are not alone on this journey. And remember, every step you take;

no matter how small, is a step towards a happier, healthier, and more fulfilled version of yourself.

*** 20 important reasons to heal our lives and free ourselves from internal emotional self-sabotage:**

Develop the ability to focus and stay on track.

2. Improve the faculties that allow us to relate better with others.

3. To free ourselves from the psychic-emotional burdens and sufferings of the past.

4. Increase our performance in all areas of our daily life.

5. Overcome the adversities that affect our temporal and spiritual progress.

6. Dilute guilt, fear, hatred, resentment, or any bad feelings.

7. Channel and channel our inner emotional self-saboteur.

8. Reprogramming our mental maps and limiting paradigms.

9. Healing our inner relationship between thoughts and emotions.

10. To strengthen our self-concept by feeling peace and inner freedom.

11. Recognize toxic "problem" people and avoid them.

12. Improve our self-esteem and strengthen our self-image.

13. To face uncertainty towards the future with determination.

14. To get in touch with our true spiritual essence.

15. Maintain a holistic balance between body and mind.

16. Establish a balance between thoughts and emotions.

17. Improve our well-being, health, lifestyle, and quality of life.

18. Generate a true and deep internal change.

19. Produce a sense of inner tranquility.

20. Healing ourselves internally.

Part Three: Learning to Transform Our Thoughts and Take Control of Them.

To apply these techniques, you must keep in mind that a negative thought, once its origin is understood, can be transmuted into positive thoughts. Similarly, limiting emotions can be transformed into more effective feelings. One of the most used tools to take control of our thoughts and emotions are empowering self-affirmations, auto-suggestion exercises, and mental auto visualization, as well as the therapies of Applied Biodescodification and

Conscious Bioneuroemotion. Techniques that allow you to channel energies, thoughts and emotions in a more adequate way and channel them for a greater good.

Let us remember that a negative thought personified by the rival black wolf attracts more negative sensations, emotions, and situations, while a positive thought in turn is greater, much stronger, and more powerful than a negative thought. So, we can channel the white wolf that represents positive thinking to attract sensations, emotions, situations, events or people with our same values and positive people who are in harmony with our principles. Because by making a shift from negative thinking to positive thinking we produce a change in our consciousness and in our mental and psychological structure, creating new realities according to the new empowered thought patterns that will allow us to completely free ourselves from that internal self-sabotage and turn it into our ally through producing a more constructive and self-directed intrapersonal conversation with oneself with a well-defined clear purpose for our progress and inner growth.

In summary, when you face a negative thought on the mental battlefield, confront it, overcome it and replace it immediately with a positive thought, you re-center your mind and channel your energies in the right direction, which will allow you to synchronize with your personal strength and power that directs our emotions and feelings resulting in a more balanced and holistic way of living allowing us to heal ourselves and enjoy better health and overall well-being.

*** The internal self-sabotage and its secret mission.**

In short, taking control of our inner warrior or white wolf to achieve success simply means facing on the battlefield the rival black wolf that dwells in every human being and defeating it. It is an exciting journey towards self-acceptance, towards the full responsibility of becoming aware of our actions and the personal enrichment that allows us to finally take control of our thoughts and emotions. The internal self-saboteur or black wolf, when analyzed in a balanced context, has very valuable aspects.

By becoming aware of our existence and channeling our influence in a positive way, we can recognize our vulnerability. This helps us to find our inner strength and rediscover the essence of our infinite power of responsibility. It allows us to take charge of our life and begin the process of inner healing.

The first step in overcoming our rival, the internal self-saboteur personified by the black wolf, is to make the decision to live and become what we really want to become. Centered on our principles and values, we choose to live in the best possible way in mental and emotional peace and harmony, both with ourselves and with our fellow human beings.

Our goal is not to completely eliminate the black wolf or internal self-saboteur, but to defeat it on the battlefield and take advantage of its valuable energy to turn it into our ally. This action will be immediately reflected and manifested in our life through the perfect synchrony between our thoughts and emotions, attracting as a result a healthier and more balanced life.

*** Final words:**

As we have learned, the power that negative emotions have in our lives through the influence of the black wolf can be limiting if we do not learn to channel them. Many people, being conditioned by them, live on autopilot generating limiting behaviors, patterns and attitudes that hinder their performance in all areas of their lives. The good news is that by realizing this internal emotional self-sabotage we can neutralize it, decoding these self-defeating behaviors and limiting subconscious programming once and for all.

The methodologies of Biodescodification and Bioneuroemotion will allow us to begin to expand our conscious mind to other dimensions of higher thoughts. At the same time, we will begin to develop a greater consciousness, finally becoming more effective and proactive people, with the capacity to solve conflicts instead of generating them.

My purpose for all of you, my reader friends, is to guide you as your personal coach so that you will never again be a prisoner of that internal emotional self-sabotage. And that through the principles of success condensed in this book you learn to change those limiting thought patterns and transform those incorrect behavioral models into more effective habits and mental programming that favor your personal growth and development.

*** The Art of Self-Transformation: How to renew, reinvent and be reborn in personal excellence.**

Personal reinvention is the courageous journey we undertake to transform our identity, beliefs, and behaviors, like an artist painting a blank canvas, consciously drawing a new image of ourselves that reflects our most authentic dreams and goals. It is a path of self-exploration and self-discovery, an intense and honest questioning of our most deeply held convictions and habits. But more than anything else, personal reinvention is an act of self-love, a determined commitment to adopt attitudes and behaviors that are aligned with our highest aspirations. Sometimes this journey begins as a response to a crisis or a major change in our lives, but it always becomes a proclamation of personal growth and development, a beacon that guides us toward realizing our fullest potential.

This journey of reinventing ourselves, of freeing ourselves from the chains of the past and emerging as transformed beings, is the essence of true liberation. It is the process that allows us to face our fears, free ourselves from our limitations and ultimately take control of our destiny.

Remember, you are the artist of your own life, and you have the ability to redraw your reality. Just as the eagle renews itself, breaking away from its old self to emerge with a new plumage, you too can reinvent yourself, renew yourself and be reborn as the phoenix from your own ashes. With every stroke of change, you are getting closer and closer to the person you really want to be. So, go ahead! Pick up the brush and start creating your new reality.

The process of reinventing yourself can be a difficult and painful journey, but the reward is priceless: the freedom to be authentically you. The beauty of this process lies in its personal and intimate nature; no one can do it for you, and no one can take away the victories you win along the way. Ultimately, personal reinvention is a path that leads to the realization of your dreams and true happiness.

* Start of our reinvestment and renewal process.

It is time for a renewal and transformation in your life. This is the beginning of a new spiritual awakening; the beginning of a new era for you. As a true peaceful warrior, you have the opportunity to heal yourself, redesign yourself and create a better version of yourself.

The alchemy of life begins when you start to die to those old structures and dream-annihilating mental schemes represented by that rival black wolf that only clung you to an uncertain past. Yes, to die to those self-sabotaging behavioral patterns and mental models that together with limiting behaviors only stopped you on your way to personal excellence.

Today you begin to take control of your life as the peaceful warrior or white wolf. You begin to heal yourself, reinvent and renew yourself as the eagle and start living large. Creating a better version of yourself where you are the sculptor, architect and builder who redesigns your own destiny and forges your own life story.

In summary, to conclude this second chapter we have learned that neither the cosmos, nor the universe, nor the stars, nor luck define your life. You build it yourself day after day. Always keep in mind that you are the main creator of your own life. You are the sculptor of your own success, the architect of your own destiny and the writer of your own story.

So go ahead! In this process of change and transformation of your being, freeing yourself from inner emotional self-sabotage in this new and exciting battle that will change your existence. Remember that this book will direct you on the path you must take, help you heal yourself and take control of your life. It will also serve as a guide to teach you how to program your mind for success and personal excellence.

However, whether you can create a new and better version of yourself is up to you. The power to heal yourself, to reinvent yourself, to be reborn as the phoenix and renewed as the eagle will depend only on you; the decision is yours. You can do it.

"Destiny may not be changed; otherwise, it would not be destiny. Man, however, can change and transform; otherwise, he would no longer be a man" - **Victor Frankl.**

"He who knows men is intelligent. He who knows himself is wise. He who overcomes others is strong. But he who overcomes himself is even stronger" - **Lao Tse.**

* The Reinvention of the Eagle: The epic of renewal.

"Nature, in its infinite wisdom and beauty, offers us numerous life lessons. Among all its creatures, one stands out in particular for its majesty and power: ***"THE EAGLE",*** *emblem of resistance and courage, whose existence is an eternal song of renewal.*

The eagle, mistress of the skies, lives longer than any other of its species, even reaching seventy years of life. However, to achieve such longevity, it must face a challenge in the middle of its life that will mark a before and after in its existence.

At the age of 40, the eagle is at a critical and delicate point. Its nails, once sharp and flexible, now long and compressed, can no longer capture prey with the same ease. Its beak, previously pointed and firm, has softened, curving against its chest, complicating hunting, and sustenance. Their wings, once powerful and light, now carry the weight of hardened and aging plumage, making it difficult for them to fly, once their greatest pride.

This eagle: faced with the crossroads, has two paths: to accept her decay and die or to embark on a painful but necessary process of renewal that will last 150 long days. If she chooses the second path, she must muster all the strength of her being, face her pain, and fly to the highest mountain, a place where solitude and hard rock will provide the shelter and protection she needs for this journey of self-transformation.

After overcoming the first obstacle, the eagle faces his next challenge. With courage and determination, he slams his beak against the rocky wall until he strips it off, in an act that borders on the sacrificial. He suffers in silence, patiently awaiting the growth of a new beak that will take weeks to emerge.

Then, the third stage of its transformation begins. With its new beak, the eagle begins to shed its old talons, tearing them off one by one, in a painful but necessary act of detachment. When its new claws emerge, robust and strong, the eagle begins the fourth and final process of its renewal.

With unwavering resolve, he begins to shed his old plumage, plucking and discarding each aging feather, making way for new, bright, and light plumage. This is the ultimate sacrifice, the last stage of his transformation that will last five long months.

When the healing and renewal process finally concludes, the eagle emerges triumphant, radiant, and more powerful than ever. Its beak renewed, its talons strengthened and its plumage shining, ready to cut through the wind and soar to the heights. After its rebirth, it takes off on the famous flight of renewal, ready to live another 30 years, full of vigor and vitality.

There, at the peak of his second life, the eagle lives his most wonderful existence, understanding that personal renewal is the true secret of his longevity. In his story, we discover a valuable lesson: like the eagle, we too can face challenges, reinvent ourselves and be reborn stronger than ever."

In our lives, there will often be times when we need to take some time out and begin our own process of healing and renewal in order to embark on our second stage towards personal excellence.

*** Points to consider:**

Personal reinvention is a decisive stage in which we have to begin the process of mental reengineering and reprogramming to start letting go of old limiting mental patterns. Freeing ourselves from internal emotional self-sabotage and releasing ourselves once and for all from the bonds of the past. Because only in this way will we be able to take advantage of the resulting benefits that a renewal always brings. And in this way, through personal reinvention we will be free, able to heal ourselves, be reborn like the phoenix, renew ourselves like the eagle and create a better version of ourselves.

There are decisive moments in our lives when we must stop and find enough courage to face the painful and difficult process of personal renewal. We must be willing to choose and make the decision that will determine the greatness of us as human beings in all the transcendental aspects of our existence. We must be decisive in life to recognize our need for a radical, total, and absolute change or transformation. Difficult times will come, different challenges and challenges that only with our renewed strength we will be able to face.

Remember that a true peaceful warrior or white wolf is one who recognizes the precise and opportune moment of a personal renewal in his life.

"I firmly believe that within each one of us there exists an authentic peaceful warrior or white wolf and there resides a vast reservoir of unlimited potentialities and competencies that usually remain dormant; waiting to be discovered and developed to blossom into our outer world. When each one of us awakens that individual potential, we will be able to face that rival black wolf and conquer our internal battles, freeing ourselves from self-sabotage, opening the way to a new conscious awakening; what I call the rebirth of the phoenix, the renewal of the eagle and personal reinvention" - **Ylich Tarazona**.

* Exercise 3: Personal renewal and reengineering process.

This third exercise of mental reengineering and reprogramming for success is intended to allow us to take the time we need to fill ourselves with courage and courage to begin our process of personal renewal as the eagle. At the same time, it allows us to decree, declare and proclaim our personal liberation by releasing us from the bonds of the past, freeing us from internal self-sabotage and any limiting thoughts or negative emotions that stop our progress. In order to be able to heal ourselves, rise from the ashes like the phoenix and create a better version of ourselves.

I decree, declare, and proclaim that today I commit myself to begin my process of personal renewal and re-engineering, freeing myself completely from everything that stops my progress in the following areas of my life...

"Doing the right things is better than doing the right things" - **Peter Drucker.**

CHAPTER III: BIOLOGICAL DECODING AND EMOTIONAL RELEASE TECHNIQUES

Introduction to the Chapter

The human being not only "has a body", but "is a body". A body formed by pure and infinite energy, condensed in molecules, atoms, electrons, neutrons, and protons. A body connected in its totality, where emotions and thoughts play a fundamental role.

Our health, well-being and quality of life depend on the knowledge we have of our body and the care we take of it. The human body has the ability to repair itself. If properly cared for, it can regain health even after injury, poisoning, infection, or other disruption.

The body's cells have the ability to regenerate, reproduce, duplicate themselves and store genetic information. If we could learn to access all this biological coding, we could prevent multiple diseases and ailments.

Part One: Biological Decoding as Alternative Therapy.

Biological decoding is a complementary technique that seeks to decipher the emotions repressed in our subconscious. Once we detect the energetic origin of an emotional conflict, biological decoding comes into play in order to reprogram the individual to solve, channel or correct the situation.

This is why biological decoding as an alternative therapy is so important, as it has been proven that repressed emotions impact our body and eventually cause symptoms, discomfort, and disease. The starting point towards wellness and fullness of life is to find those moments in which a person has suffered a strong level of stress in their life, imbalance or emotional shock and recognize the situation that caused that stress or energetic imbalance that has been anchored in the body.

Once we find the trigger that is causing the imbalance, it is easier to undertake a subjective path of healing from the biological decoding. It is necessary to understand that before presenting a manifest disease, in most cases the human being goes through a process of stress or traumatic event. This situation later becomes significant and is the main cause of the appearance of symptoms or any other ailment.

The subject having lived or experienced some conflict creates a biological action that can manifest a symbolic meaning in the face of that unexpected situation, producing in many cases a disease. This unresolved biological conflict or the one that we did not manage to heal at the time tends to remain anchored within the body or organism. Subsequently, when remaining stagnant in the organism, with the time the same body begins to express externally some symptom.

It is enough to observe the experiences, problematic situations, interpersonal or emotional conflicts of human beings to see how these circumstances generate a strong stress that eventually produces the palpable appearance of some symptom or disease in the individual. This is where biological decoding can be used as an alternative therapy to begin a process of energetic balance and emotional healing.

It is important to emphasize at this point that biological decoding or Biodecoding does not replace medical or psychological treatments, but rather complements them. And to complement this healing process, the Biodecoding tries to find the emotional and energetic meaning of the diseases caused by some kind of emotions (negative feelings and thoughts) that are not manifested as such and that for that reason are projected in the physical plane of the body manifesting themselves through some symptom or disease.

Keep in mind that this manifestation is an approximation of what is related to the diseases and has no diagnostic value in itself. Each person is unique and, therefore, so is their way of physically expressing their emotions. However, as human beings we share the biological, collective, and symbolic meaning of our organs and systems, as well as the same molecular formation and structure. So, there are certain genetic patterns that tend to repeat themselves from generation to generation.

Health is the most precious and invaluable asset we possess and is about who we are and what we do. It is vital both to preserve it and to seek healing when it is threatened by disease, illness, symptom, or disturbing emotion.

Having the ability to take charge of our health will not only allow us to take care of it, but also to prevent illnesses before they appear or manifest.

*** The practical application of biological decoding in daily life can begin with the following steps:**

1. **Self-awareness**: Begin to pay attention to the emotional patterns and physical responses that occur in response to stressful life events. When do physical symptoms appear? What emotions are you experiencing at the time? Taking note of these connections can help you identify patterns in your life.

Acknowledgement: Identify and accept the emotions and thoughts that arise, rather than ignoring or repressing them. Take time each day to reflect on your emotions and experiences. You don't have to judge them or change them; simply acknowledge them.

3. **Emotional expression**: Instead of repressing your emotions, find ways to express them. This may involve talking about your emotions with a trusted friend, writing in a journal, art therapy, meditation or talk therapy.

4. **Self-care**: Maintain a healthy diet, exercise regularly and get enough sleep. These factors can contribute to better emotional and physical health.

5. **Professional help**: If you feel that repressed emotions are significantly affecting your life, seek the help of a professional. Biological decoding therapists can provide specific tools and strategies to help you release repressed emotions and heal your emotional conflicts.

6. **Emotional support**: Seek support from loved ones and close friends. Don't be afraid to ask for help when you need it. Your loved ones can provide you with the strength and motivation you need to overcome your emotional challenges.

7. **Continuous learning**: Continue to learn and grow emotionally. Biological decoding is a journey, not a destination. Continue to develop your emotional skills and look for new ways to improve your emotional well-being.

8. **Practice mindfulness**: Relaxation, Breathing, Meditation and Mindfulness or mindfulness will help you maintain focus on the present, which is essential in biological decoding. Practice mindfulness techniques such as meditation and yoga.

9. **Forgiveness**: Forgiveness can be an important step in releasing repressed emotions. Learning to forgive others and you can be a powerful step toward healing and emotional balance.

Remember that biological decoding is a personal process, and each individual has his or her own pace and needs. It is essential to be patient and compassionate with yourself throughout this journey of self-exploration and healing.

Part Two: Knowing Our Emotions

*** Fear as a manifest symptom.**

Fear is a primary emotion represented by the black wolf that manifests itself when the person interprets a situation as dangerous. The reactions of this rival can be to flee, to attack, to defend oneself, etc. Its function is the survival of the species. The first emotional regulation to overcome fear is confidence represented by the white wolf.

*** Strategies to regulate fear and control inner self-sabotage.**

Self-reflection questions that can help identify, accept, and regulate fear. Trusting oneself and others is the primary emotional regulation for overcoming and mastering fear. Here are some strategies to improve self-confidence and foster confidence in others.

1. Review your internal dialogue (inner voice) in fearful situations. What do you say to yourself? Use positive language with yourself and others. Acknowledge the presence of fear (black wolf), accept it, and maintain conscious communication and redirect the emotion with positive thoughts and feelings.

2. Formulate the objectives in a positive way, divide them into small challenges that are achievable and that depend on oneself.

3. To build self-confidence, put the focus on the task you want to do and then start executing a step-by-step action plan. That is, the first step you need to take to achieve your goals is to break down your responsibilities into small challenges. Then focus your efforts on achieving those small goals one after another in order of priority with a set date. The consecutive achievement of those small challenges will eventually allow us to achieve the expected final goal at the end of the set deadline. In summary, start with an end in mind (clear objective), then break it down into small challenges, set a deadline to follow and begin the process of achieving each small goal one at a time until the desired end goal is reached.

4. Avoid setting your expectations too high in the beginning, start small and build up as you become stronger, more confident, and secure.

5. Regularly review your action plan and make sure you are on track. According to what you have planned, regularly evaluate what you are achieving and keep in mind what needs to be improved.

6. Learn to recognize the positive things in yourself and others. Recognizing the good qualities in yourself and others is a form of self-recognition and, therefore, a source of self-confidence.

7. See mistakes as a lesson: every mistake is a steppingstone to your success if you learn from it, accept it, and ask yourself what you can do next time to improve. Learn from your past experiences. Remember that without mistakes there is no learning and no improvement.

8. Connect with past experiences that were positive: bringing to mind the small and big accomplishments you have achieved allows you to connect and anchor that experience in a more empowered way. Try to remember how you felt and acted: see, feel, and hear what you experienced in that past experience and bring those good emotions and thoughts into the present.

*** Sadness: strategies to overcome this emotion.**

Sadness is an emotion felt when a person interprets a situation as a loss. Like the previous ones, this emotion is a manifestation of the black wolf. The reaction is to feel despondency, the desire to cry and isolate oneself. The function of sadness is cohesion and the emotional regulation to channel it correctly is to comfort this sadness.

Ask yourself the following questions and answer them as sincerely and honestly as possible: *What makes me sad? Where do I feel the discomfort? How does this situation make me feel? What are the consequences of this situation for me? What is hurting me? What is not helping me find comfort? What am I not accepting? What is making me sad? How can I comfort this sadness? What am I becoming aware of? What can I learn from this emotion?*

1. Being aware of what you feel, where you feel and how you express it is the first step in taking control of the situation.

2. Allow yourself to express this emotion through crying when necessary. Crying is a good way to let off steam and release that stagnant emotion if it is done as an emotional release therapy and not as a repetitive habit.

3. Sadness is an emotion that can be confused with anger. A sadness that is not properly regulated or that is not given the space to cry and release it in a healthy way can end up generating anger.

*** Rabies: some strategies for healthy responses.**

Anger is a primary emotion that is felt when a person interprets a situation as unfair. Rage is another manifestation of the black wolf and is a rival that is good to keep under control. The reaction of rage is to attack hitting, shouting, insulting, etc. Your function to use it to your advantage is to generate changes and emotional regulation is to manifest that emotion, recognize it and channel it in a better way. Allow your white wolf to take control of the situation.

*** Strategies to regulate anger.**

Self-reflection questions that can help identify, accept, and regulate (channel) anger: let this emotion out through constructive activities that allow it to be channeled more effectively with activities that suit the preferences of each person, situation, and environment. For example:

1. Do sports or other physical exercise activities that help you to drain that emotion in a healthier way.

2. Write down everything you feel: you can put down on paper your feelings, unburden yourself, writing and then tear up and throw that paper away.

3. Contact a trusted person or therapist who will listen to your experience and your feelings without judgment and help you channel that emotion into a correct and liberating path.

*** Other strategies to regulate rabies are:**

- Move away from the situation that produces the anger, if possible.

- Check your inner voice, i.e., what do I say to myself in this situation? Send yourself positive messages such as: Relax, everything will be fine, what can I do next time to avoid this situation?

- Divert attention to another, more pleasant issue.

- Once the person is calmer, they can examine how they feel about the particular situation and ask themselves what can I do so that on another similar occasion they can respond in a more positive way?

- Become aware of the cause: with whom does it happen to me, in what situations, is it frequent or repetitive? Keep in mind that if the situation is not addressed or put aside, the feelings will not go away.

- If you react intuitively instead of giving a more responsible and mature response to the situation, you should ask yourself questions such as: What are my options besides getting upset, is this situation bad enough to get on my nerves?

- Take situations in stride: sometimes it is easy to take minor problems too seriously.

- These strategies need more time, effort, and training, but the goal is emotional regulation and education in the face of anger.

- Be aware of the initial warning signs in order to act before reaching the emotional outburst. These signs can be strong heartbeat, tension in the chest or jaw, feelings of resentment, irritation, among others.

- Talk to someone you trust (therapist) who can help assess situations more clearly, as reactivity may be a sign of another unresolved problem.

- When the circumstances that generate anger, such as job loss, separation, illness, etc., cannot be controlled. You can see what strategies other people in similar situations are developing to manage these same situations more successfully.

- Learning strategies on healthy thinking, problem solving, conflict management, enhancing self-esteem and "assertiveness" allows to manage emotions in a better way.

- Practice healthy habits in daily life activities such as: eating, sleeping and physical exercise.

- If you feel frustrated when others do not act as you wish, it is important to remember that you cannot control the behaviors of others. You can only control your own behaviors and your own reactions to these behaviors.

- These strategies do not solve the problem that originates the anger, but they give the person the ability to take control over the situation and decide what response he/she wants to give to the current circumstance.

- Count to 10. Breathe deeply by taking abdominal breaths.

*** Shame and how to overcome it:**

Shame is a secondary emotion also represented by this black wolf adversary. This feeling is felt when the person interprets a situation by making a moral judgment about him/herself that is not consistent with his/her personal values. The reaction is reddening, feeling of failure, desire to hide or shyness. Its function is to generate internal conscience and the emotional regulation to channel it correctly is to forgive and accept oneself.

*** Strategies to regulate embarrassment:**

Self-reflection questions that can help identify, accept, and regulate shame effectively:

- What is my opinion of myself?
- How does this situation make me feel?
- What am I saying to myself?
- What label have I put on?
- What is the most embarrassing thing about this situation?
- What am I avoiding expressing?
- What image do I want to project?
- What do I not accept about myself?
- How am I judging myself?
- What am I ashamed of?
- What behavior do I want to improve?
- What do I need to accept?
- What do I need to forgive myself?
- What do I need to free myself from?
- What am I becoming aware of?

What can be done in the face of one's own and others' shame:

- Be aware of what you feel, where you feel it and how it is expressed.
- Be aware of the labels and moral judgments that people make or the labels we make about ourselves.
- To be able to forgive ourselves when we are not up to the task, and we have let ourselves down.
- Understanding that perfection does not exist and accepting who we are is the way to take control of the situation.
- When you acquire the competence to forgive yourself, you can begin to forgive others.

*** Guilt and how to release it correctly:**

Guilt is a secondary emotion and like the previous ones is represented by the black wolf. It manifests itself when the person interprets an experience in which he/she has made a mistake or error. The reaction is to control the damage, disapproval, "I should have done...", etc. Its function is to generate external awareness. The emotional regulation to release it is learning, acceptance and love.

*** Strategies to Release Guilt:**

Questions that allow us to become aware and begin the process of emotional liberation:

- What mistake have I made in this situation? And what do I need to repair?

- How does this situation make me feel?

- How does it make me feel to have made a mistake?

- What consequences has my mistake had for other people?

- Where did I go wrong? And how can I best correct it?

- Who do I think I have failed? And how can I make restitution?

- What are the implications of this mistake at this point in my life?

- What do I think I should have done?

- How do I feel about not having been able to control it?

- What do I need to repair? Or what do I need to verify?

- What am I learning from this situation?

- How do I feel about learning from this situation? And what does this learning allow me to do?

- What am I becoming aware of?

*** What can be done in the face of one's own and others' guilt:**

- Be aware of what you feel, where you feel it and how it is expressed.

- Once guilt has been identified, the empowering questions that allow to regulate this guilt are:

What do I need to learn from this situation? And what do I need to learn about myself?

- Apologizing sincerely allows us to make amends and enables us to avoid committing the same situations on another occasion, helping us to avoid committing the same incident again.

- Feeling regret honestly enables people to repair the wrong done and avoid committing it again on future occasions.

- Learning from the situation and not making the same mistake again prevents us from feeling guilty and frees us from guilt.

*** The power of love:**

Love is a primary emotion that is felt when the person interprets an experience as an offering and is represented by the WHITE WOLF. The reaction is fullness, ecstasy, serenity, passion, charity, and its function are transcendence. Emotional regulation is the just correspondence of this love. Although in this model love is considered a primary emotion, there are other authors who consider it a secondary or derived emotion.

*** Strategies to regulate love:**

Self-reflection questions that can help to identify, accept, and regulate love:

- What can I give in this reaction? And what do I receive in return?

- How does this situation make me feel?

- What is it costing me to receive? Or what do I need to give?

- What is the universe not giving me back?

- What are you rejecting? Or what am I rejecting?

- What evaluation do I receive from myself? And what evaluation do I receive from others?

- How do I express my love? And what proofs of love do I receive?

- What is this situation offering me? And what am I offering to this situation?

- What am I giving to myself? And what can I offer to the universe?

- What do I feel when I give love to myself? And what do I feel when I receive it?

- What am I becoming aware of? And what should I learn about love?

*** What can be done about the love we feel, and the love felt by others:**

- Being aware of what we feel, where we feel it and how we express it.

- Love always needs correspondence. This can be expressed in many ways: with material or intangible details, expression of mutual feelings, feeling good about something done or received, etc.

- Love is present in action and manifests itself in many ways through the simplest details of life.

- It is important to be attentive to the proofs of love, gestures of genuine affection that are received or given between one person to another. For this is the most ideal way to offer and receive love. And, therefore, the best way in which love manifests itself.

- The intensity with which proofs of love are given and received must also be in harmony between the parties. For if more is received than is given or if more is given than is received, there is no correct regulation of this emotion.

- In terms of gender, men, and women express love in different ways. Generally, women need small daily acknowledgments and men need big acknowledgments, but not as often.

*** Joy: an emotion that is transmitted:**

Joy is a primary emotion that is felt when the person interprets an experience as a gain and is represented by the WHITE WOLF. The reaction is to jump, to love, to sing, euphoria, happiness, ecstasy, etc. Its function is the facilitation and emotional regulation is to be able to share it, express it and spread it in a positive way.

*** Questions to consider:**

- How does this situation make me feel? And what am I gaining from this situation?

- With whom do I want to share my joy? And what is preventing me from sharing it?

- What challenge have I overcome? And what satisfies me the most?

- What makes me happier? And what do I want to celebrate?

- How will I share it, and what does it say about me?

- What am I becoming aware of?

*** How joy manifests itself:**

- Joy needs to be shared with others in order to be able to regulate this emotion well.

- When joy cannot be shared openly, it can generate discomfort.

- It is important to create situations that allow us to live and experience moments of joy.

- It is vitally important to give and receive joy. For this is a healing and very liberating emotion.

Part Three: Energetic therapeutic writing to decode emotional problems:

Therapeutic writing exercises to decode emotional problems that affect your health. If you are worried about a problem that is affecting you emotionally or affects your body energetically, I recommend you try to practice emotional writing. To do this I propose these exercises writing for about 21 minutes, over 7 days.

Concentrate on the situation that is affecting you. The most crucial thing is that when you write, you do it without stopping and without taking into account grammatical or syntactical rules. Because only then will you be able to give free rein to what you feel. Remember that this is a writing exercise of emotional liberation, not a literary, grammatical, or orthographic work.

*** First Exercise:**

The objective is simply to write about your innermost thoughts and feelings related to the event that is affecting you. Just explore the event in question and write about how it has affected you. As you progress in therapeutic writing you can begin to link that event to other aspects of your life.

Ask yourself how that emotion is linked to your childhood, to your parents or to people who have played an important role in your life. You should ask yourself how that discomfort is related to your current life and what role it might play in your future. The idea is to look for links between that event and your past. You should also find a relationship to the person you have become and the person you would like to be in the future.

*** Second Exercise:**

On the second day you should delve even deeper into your feelings and thoughts to assess the effect they have had on the different spheres of your life. Evaluate how your reaction or response to the event may have affected or benefited you and try to determine to what extent you were responsible for what happened.

Keep in mind that this exercise is not about going on a witch hunt in search of culprits, but rather understanding your level of responsibility so that you do not make the same mistakes again in the future. Remember that learning from our mistakes makes us wiser.

*** Third Exercise:**

The time has come to start looking ahead. In those 21 minutes of writing, you should explore the situation from different points of view. That is, try to assume a more rational perspective as if you were an outside observer. You can put yourself in the shoes of different people and think about how they would view the situation you are concerned about. It is also important that you write about the points that make you more vulnerable to adversity, so you learn to know yourself better.

* **Fourth Exercise**:

On the fourth day you should reflect on everything you have written. Review your notes and assess if there are any issues that you have overlooked. Reflect on what you have learned and gained from this experience. Write it down. It is also important to reflect on how this event has shaped your behavior and how it might help you in the future.

* **Fifth Exercise**:

On this fifth day, finish writing a short story as if it were a short story in which you include the situation you experienced. Make sure it has a happy, positive, and encouraging ending that motivates and inspires you to move forward with firmness and determination despite the adversities. In this way, you will be able to make sense of all the aspects related to that painful experience and by giving it a happy and positive ending, you allow the current situation to lose its negative emotional impact and become a more pleasant experience. You will have modified its original meaning and anchored a desired emotional state. This technique in NLP or neurolinguistic programming is called anchor collapse, due to the fact that it generates a new, more empowered neural groove in relation to that same experience. By modifying it in the story, the actual situation in your brain, memory and neurons is also modified.

Before continuing with the sixth and seventh exercises, I will share with you some tips to get the most out of this therapeutic writing therapy. *What should you keep in mind when practicing expressive writing?* To get the most out of this technique, you should keep in mind that some forms of writing are more beneficial than others. Therefore, you should follow these five basic principles:

1. Write about the negative events that disturb you and that you do not want to tell anyone else and write them on a sheet of paper. Keep in mind that this exercise is personal and only you will see the content of the sheets you write.

2. Properly identify the emotions you experience, both negative and positive. And accept them because in this way you will learn to release the energetic charges that produce those emotions in your organism.

3. Construct a coherent and meaningful story that includes the situation that affects you. Then turn the story around and create an ending where you are

victorious over the situation that is empowering, motivating, and inspiring to you.

4. Narrate the facts from different perspectives using different pronouns, this way you will be able to cover different points of view. Remember to be creative in capturing everything you feel, see, and hear. Make the therapeutic writing technique a multisensory activity.

5. Do not censor any thoughts. It is important that you write with sincerity, but at the same time try not to use the exercise to protest or regret, on the contrary, use the exercise to accept those emotions, thoughts, and situations, learn from them and make the most of them.

To continue with the next two exercises, pay attention to the indications: It is of vital importance that before proceeding to exercises 6 and 7 you must have performed the first 5 previous exercises. If you have already done the previous exercises, then let's move on to perform these two new therapeutic writing techniques called captain of your soul, which consists of doing the writing and in addition to that do other actions together to get the most out of it. To do this just follow the instructions step by step and ready, so without further ado let's go with the therapeutic writing exercises called "**Captain of your Soul**".

*** Sixth Exercise**:

Take a piece of paper and a pen and write down everything you don't like in your life. Give yourself permission in this therapeutic exercise to bring out the judgmental side that we all carry inside and write down on the paper everything that you dislike, that makes you uncomfortable and that you do not agree with currently in your life.

Step 1: Try to express in each sentence the anger and frustration that this negative situation makes you feel. Try to express it by reflecting all that you carry inside and that you normally would not express to anyone else. Write it all down on that paper, don't leave anything out. Remember that this is a personal therapeutic writing exercise, very intimate and private. That no one is going to look at or read, because at the end I will show you the right way to get rid of that piece of paper. So be confident and write whatever you feel and whatever crosses your mind, no matter how intimate it is, because only you will see it. You simply write on the paper everything you don't like about your life trying to express the anger, disappointment, despair, or negative feeling it makes you feel.

Step number 2: Once you have finished writing down what you don't like about your life, now look at that piece of paper where you have written everything that makes you feel so bad and ask yourself how do you feel when you look at this piece of paper? Naturally, you will answer me that you feel bad, full of anger or frustration, maybe it turns your stomach, that's fine, this is normal for this part of the exercise. Now to continue I ask you; don't you feel like breaking all these things in your life? Yes, don't you feel like tearing up this paper and what it represents? Then crumple it, crumple it, tear it, bite it, shred it, tear it, tear it to pieces, tear it apart and destroy that piece of paper.

Once you are done with this step, we are going to continue with the next decisive step to free yourself from those emotions and energetic charges. Now let's burn the paper, okay, let's burn all this negative stuff! You can do it with caution in a bathroom, a sink or somewhere that is ventilated and safe. The first thing you should do is burn the paper inside a large cooking pot so that it is safe and also the ashes are deposited inside the pot. The more it will go, the more liberating it will be to burn the paper and the blacker smoke will come out. The more blackness that paper represents, the more liberating it will be to burn. For this reason, I encourage you to burn the paper completely and watch closely as the paper burns and smolders, visualize how the smoke carries away your worries, see how the fire consumes the paper as you feel how you begin to free yourself from those negative emotions. As the paper burns to ashes the more and more liberated you will feel.

Once you see the paper burn and you see it turn into ashes, throw those ashes that are deposited in the pot being careful not to burn yourself, be sure to throw those ashes down the drain of your W.C. toilet, bathroom, or toilet bowl if you are inside the house. The important thing is that it is a place where there is plenty of water flowing to carry everything away safely. The most valuable thing is to watch carefully how the water carries away the ashes and imagine how it also carries away your energetic charges.

Feel, think, visualize, and imagine how both the fire that destroys the paper and the water that discards the ashes represent your liberation. The burning paper symbolically represents purification. Watching the leaves burn represents letting go of whatever must leave your life. Just as the smoke ascends, so too does it let all negative emotions flow freely. The water, on the other hand, represents cleansing as watching the ashes go down the drain you have used for the exercise symbolically represents liberation.

Step 3: Once you have done the previous steps, go back to the table or whatever place you are using to do the Therapeutic Writing Exercise. Take a few seconds to feel that liberating process. How do you feel right now? How therapeutic and liberating did you find the exercise? How good do you feel now that you have symbolically freed yourself from all those energetic charges that were affecting your emotional health? This makes you feel liberated, doesn't it? And you feel much better now, don't you? You will see that you certainly feel much better now. Mentally answering these questions is important, as it generates a positive neural reconversion within you. By admitting that you are feeling better inside with the therapeutic writing therapy, new neuronal grooves will be created in your mind and a synapse will be produced in your neurons creating a new sensation of emotional liberation. This is called mental reprogramming in NLP. This reprogramming will help your subconscious subjectively accept the release and, therefore, the writing therapy becomes even more effective.

*** Seventh Exercise**:

Now to continue we are going to take another sheet of paper and in this seventh and last exercise we are going to write down all the good things for which you feel grateful.

Step 1: We are going to write down on this new sheet of paper a list of all the things you are grateful for. You are going to write down at least 21 things, situations, or people for which you are grateful. To help you recognize those 21 things, situations, or people for which you are grateful you can help yourself with the following questions: What do you have in your life for which you can be grateful? Remember that we all have thousands of events for which we can be grateful, but which we usually overlook. A man once said I was worried because I had no shoes until I saw a man who had no feet. So, what things do you have for which you can be thankful? Find them all and write them down on paper. Do you have health? Write down I am thankful that I am in good health. So, what is it that you do have? For example, do you have two arms? Two legs? A head? So, you are alive, and you have health, write it down on a piece of paper! Even if you're missing a couple of limbs, you'll find that you still have many others for which you're thankful. Do you have eyes? Ears? Then write it down on paper! Maybe you don't yet realize how much that's worth! Now, what else do you have? Do you have a roof to sleep under? And in that house, you live in, do you have people who love you? Who are they? Do you love them too? Then write down on the paper: A home full of people who love me. Do you realize what a treasure all this is?

Write down the name of each of those jewels you own! How? Simply ask yourself: who are those people who love you? perhaps your partner? and do you love them with all your heart? then write their name on the paper! Is there anyone else? perhaps your children? or your parents? write their names on the paper? and friends? do you have friends? do you have friends? write their names on the paper? do you believe in God? do you consider that he loves you? if so, write them down too! Write their names down on the paper! What about friends? Do you have friends? Write their names down on the paper! Do you believe in God? Do you consider that he loves you? If so, then write that down on the paper too! What about your values? Do you possess integrity? Are you an honest and upright person? If so, then write it down on the paper! Do you have access to something special in your life? Of course, you do! You're doing this exercise, aren't you? Write it down too! What other treasures do you have in your life? Think about them! Find them and write them down! And what else? Do you live in a beautiful place? Do you love your land? If so, write it down on your paper: the beautiful land of my ancestors.

Step number 2: Open the window and look up at the sky, what do you see? the sky! Look down a little bit, what is it, the earth! Do you realize, you live on planet earth! You have this whole huge planet to enjoy, so write down on the paper: a beautiful planet to live on and be happy. If you have any other treasures, write them down on the paper and you will see that you have many.

Step 3: Now stand up. Look at the paper and read it out loud. What do you see? Your life is full of treasures! Do you realize it? Many times, we don't take them into account, but you have to look at them because they are all the good things we have now, they are all the reasons to be happy and there are many of them! So be sure to write down on paper, all the things that you are grateful for. When you have a good list with at least 21 things you are grateful for.

Step number 4: Look at your piece of paper, read it again and recognize that you have many things written on it for which to be grateful. Keep in mind that we all have many things to be grateful for in this life, even if we don't consciously think about them. How do you feel when you look at that piece of paper? You feel good and grateful, don't you? At this moment you feel happy, joyful, excited to do the exercise. Right?

Excellent we have finished the 7 therapeutic writing exercises. Congratulations, it feels wonderful, doesn't it?

These techniques are one of the most powerful ways to free ourselves from that inner emotional self-sabotage and feed the WHITE WOLF, allowing this inner warrior to take control of our life.

*** The magic scenario.**

The objective of the technique is to unblock the negative thought processes of the brain. These processes usually occur after experiencing experiences with a strong emotional charge, emotional charges that keep the brain looking for solutions to the problem within the limits of limiting thought that prevent it from seeking solutions to the conflict in question. However, the technique consists of imagining how we would solve the problem if we had magical powers. Imagining that we possess magical powers makes it easier for the subconscious brain to explore new creative solutions and gradually relax its stagnant state.

Imagine that you are a superhero or heroine, a person with extraordinary gifts that allow you to solve any adversity or challenge, no matter how difficult it may seem. By imagining that you have these mystical and super heroic qualities, it allows you to see the problem from another perspective. Since the brain relaxes, it enters a more favorable state and releases all the tension of having to look for a solution in a traditional way.

Let's remember that for the brain it is the same to imagine, visualize and interpret what happens in a symbolic or figurative way, without having the ability to recognize if an action is real or created (imagined). So, your brain will look for unimaginable solutions that you thought impossible before.

Step Number 1: One of the ways to apply this technique would be to remember the conflict situation and visualize or imagine it as if you were watching it from a movie screen. Once the mental image has originated as a movie, enter the scene with the characters frozen in time. Magically fix all the details of the problem (remember, everything has a solution, you are a magician or superhero or heroine). Be creative, let your creativity fly and let all your ideas flow without question. Write down everything you can think of.

You can repeat the process several times and you will see how the solutions will change. Ask yourself: How can I do it differently this time? Make all the modifications you think are necessary and imagine several scenarios where you manage to overcome the adversities. Focus your attention on all the alternatives and options you can think of to improve the story of your movie. Now, take a deep breath, step out of the movie, and see how it flows with the changes you have made.

Step Number 2: Repeat the previous steps, but this time exaggerating the situation a bit more. Use your magic potions and use your superpowers with increasing confidence until you feel that the situation is no longer a problem. Visualize and imagine your movie having managed to come out of the situation victorious again. Feel how you feel at that moment, listen to what you would say to yourself and pay attention to what you hear from people congratulating you on your great deed. See what you have accomplished, contemplate your results, and imagine how happy you must be feeling.

This NLP technique is known as creative visualization and is combined with several other NLP techniques such as: Visual Power Scenario, Association or Dissociation and Anchor Collapse. What makes this technique so powerful is that it employs the "submodalities" and sensory representations (sight/what we see, hearing/what we hear and kinesthetic/what we feel and experience). That is, each of the sensory qualities that we differentiate in what is detected by the different channels of perception through our five senses. For the visual channel we would have color, brightness, size, movement, angle of vision, shape, etc. For the auditory channel: tempo, tone, volume, rhythm, timbre, origin, etc. And for the kinesthetic channel (touch, smell, taste): pressure, location, extension, temperature, movement, etc.

By modifying these submodalities in our mind, we are forcing the subconscious to generate an internal change in what we perceive of the real situation, according to what we imagine. Performing this creative visualization exercise is important since it generates a positive neuronal reconversion within you. As you imagine different situations where you use your magical faculties or superpowers to solve those problems in a creative way, new neuronal grooves will be created in your mind. And a synapse will be produced in your neurons, producing a new sensation of emotional liberation. What in NLP is called mental reprogramming.

This reprogramming will help your subconscious to subjectively seek solutions to real life adversities. And, therefore, creative visualization therapy becomes even more effective, as it allows you to see whatever challenges you are going through in your real life from a much more positive perspective.

Part Four: Healing with the practice of Ho'oponopono.

Ho'oponopono allows us to channel negative thoughts and limiting emotions, allowing us to regain inner peace. Meet this ancient Hawaiian technique, ideal for the solution and dissolution of worries. The term Ho'oponopono means "to correct a mistake" and gives its name to a philosophy of life that comes from Hawaii. It is based on a process of recognition, repentance, forgiveness, love, gratitude, and transmutation. Emotions that allow a mental cleansing of limiting thoughts and negative feelings to eliminate energetic blockages and regain inner peace.

This millenary Hawaiian technique holds that the subject who practices it is in connection with God, the universe, the infinite universal source, and is responsible for what happens to him/her. It does not seek to blame others or circumstances and considers that the solutions to any evil, whether physical or psychological, are precisely within each person. It is about becoming aware that we are responsible for the emotions we experience when faced with the problems and situations we live.

Through Ho'oponopono, harmful memories or emotional imbalances, whether conscious or subconscious, are cleared and a sense of release from worries is obtained. There are many ways to use this technique: as long as responsibility, love, forgiveness, gratitude and recognition are protagonists, we are performing Ho'oponopono.

Here you will see a concrete protocol: establish and investigate the cause of a problem or situation you wish to improve or correct. State, out loud or under your breath, that you are going to perform a Ho'oponopono process. State what the problem or situation is that you want to work on. Remember that recognizing the conflict allows us to accept it and therefore it is easier to release it and let it flow. Ask for the collaboration of the subconscious mind and the superconscious mind.

Investigate your relationship with that problem and become aware of the situation with these types of questions: *what is in me that can cause or be related to this situation or problem, what internal memories are related, what patterns and behaviors do I repeat that I can improve, how do I behave in front of that problem or situation, how can I solve it, what do I think about the issue, how do I feel about that situation, how do I feel about that situation, how do I feel about that situation?*

Is there related anger, fear, guilt? Or, on the contrary, is there love, acceptance, forgiveness, and gratitude? What can I do to improve the situation? Write down all your findings in a notebook. Become aware of your behaviors on a mental, emotional, and spiritual level.

*** Attitudes for Ho'oponopono:**

Whenever you do Ho'oponopono you should consider, at every moment, these aspects: Inspiration: While reflecting or cleansing, you should always be open to listen to the information that inspiration gives you. Perhaps a memory comes to mind, an emotional association, an awareness of a pattern of behavior you repeat, or something you have often wished for. Much of this information will be within your conscious grasp when you raise the issue, while much of it will surface as inspiration during the process.

Regret: Take responsibility for having accepted a series of patterns, beliefs, memories, and emotional associations that are related to the problem we are dealing with. Take responsibility for the emotions that you have had to maintain and become aware of the emotions that you have to transform. Be aware that everything in your life is created through your memories (thoughts, feelings, emotions, and actions). Nothing in your reality is incompatible with them. Whenever you are aware of a wrong memory, pattern, or behavior, you must understand that you should not have done it (although we all have the right to make mistakes, we also have the power to correct them). To the point of deciding that you would never go back and never repeat it again. Choose another better behavior that is more appropriate or choose the method to learn how to behave better in the same situation.

Repair: Whenever you become aware of an incorrect action or way of thinking or feeling, you must correct the mistake from your conscious mind. If you caused harm, recognize your mistake, abandon excuses, ask for forgiveness and try to repair or restore the damage. If your way of acting, feeling and thinking are not the best, write down how you would like to do it and look for ways to learn to do it better.

*** Point to consider:**

If you become aware of a wrong behavior or a way of thinking or feeling that you need to improve and you consciously decide to do nothing (i.e., continue with the mistake), then the Ho'oponopono exercise will do you no good. For, if you simply repeat the phrases, mantras, or prayers for the inner divinity to change everything for you, nothing will happen. Your inner divinity will never force you to make a change if you consciously choose to persist in doing nothing about it. So first decide what changes you will need to make and what behaviors you will need to learn. Reflect on how you will ask for forgiveness and be prepared to love and forgive.

Balance: Trust in the process, trust in the basic selves that depend on you and trust in that higher and infinite universal force that is also working and doing its part. If the conscious mind has its collaboration, you will be able to transform your behaviors, patterns, and beliefs much more easily. You have to be willing to forgive, love and release. Give up demanding reparation if you have been hurt, because if you expect something in return you remain attached to the problem instead of releasing.

*** Steps to perform a Ho'oponopono exercise:**

Step Number 1: Relaxation and breathing. Now you are going to start the actual cleansing with the mantra (I'm sorry, I'm sorry, thank you, I love you). Find a comfortable position and repeat this mantra (I recommend using slow, controlled breathing while repeating the following mantra). Assuming you already know Ho'oponopono and the four phrases (sorry, sorry, thank you, I love you), simply repeat the four statements over and over again as you imagine, hear and feel them. So, you can simply sit and concentrate. You can say them out loud or in your mind as you want to use them.

This Hawaiian technique of these four phrases has impacted the lives of many people over the years, so let it impact yours as well. So, without further ado, let's start with the exercise: I'm sorry. Please forgive me. Thank you. I love you. I am sorry. Please, please, please forgive me. Thank you. I love you. I love you. I love you. I'm sorry. I'm sorry. Please, please forgive me. I love you. I love you. I love you. I'm sorry. I'm sorry. Please forgive me. Thank you. I love you. I love you. I love you.

I hope you enjoyed this Ho'oponopono mantra. You are now ready to free yourself and move on to step number two.

Step Number 2: Dialogue with the mind to connect it with the power of Ho'oponopono. Become aware that the mind accepted or created a memory stored in the subconscious and that this stored memory is the creative source of a past, present, or future situation. The conscious mind cannot always fully know these memories; however, these memories are recorded in the subconscious mind.

Ask the subconscious mind, with love and humility, to raise the request to clear your memories to the inner divinity, maintaining the charge of vital energy through the breath. Now you know that the supra conscious mind (a higher state of consciousness) participates in the liberation process. This supra-conscious state allows us to evaluate memories and can send us inspirations and flashes of intuition.

Remain open to change and the flow of healing energy. Be attentive to the inspiration and flashes of intuition that will help you erase those stagnant memories and emotions and release them.

Step Number 3: Change your vision. Whenever you feel you are stuck in the process and wish to move forward, try the following: talk to the things, situations and body parts involved with the situation you intend to improve or correct. Thank them for their involvement in your life, especially if they also suffer in response to your memories.

Consider that people, although they are beings of light connected to the same divine and universal source, like all human beings, can generate suffering, do wrong and sometimes absurd things. Therefore, cultivating love, forgiveness, and a true sincere desire to forget are the best qualities to overcome any memory that has affected us in some way or another.

Apologize to things, situations, and people for the damage you have unintentionally caused them. Express your desire to change your patterns and your conviction that improvement is possible. Listen again to inspiration and let yourself be guided. Ask for learning to take place for the transformation of these memories. Learn to release others so that you can be released as well. Let go of past memories so that the world, people and things can show you, their perfection.

Step Number 4: Stay focused with the 4 initial phrases (sorry, sorry, thank you, I love you). The longer the practice lasts, the better results you will get. After all of the above it is interesting to keep the attention of the conscious mind in the releasing process, without doing anything else but being present in the here and now.

As you make it a habit to repeat the four phrases, the more they will become familiar in your subconscious and the more they will become part of your inner being. As you perform the mantra of the four power phrases (sorry, sorry, thank you, I love you) try to make sense to yourself and connect with the emotions that each of them represents.

In ancient Hawaiian traditions the number 108 is said to have healing and liberating power when repeating the power phrases (sorry, sorry, thank you, I love you). So, once you get more practice in conscious breathing, meditation, and concentration, the easier it will be to repeat the mantra 108 times in a row in the same liberation session. When you achieve this, you will see how you will feel more and more liberated from those memories of the past that had been anchored.

To finish the exercise, repeat the mantra. This time with a higher level of awareness than the previous one, paying attention to your breathing and keeping your concentration in the here and now.

"I am sorry. Please forgive me. Thank you. I love you." This is a powerful mantra that you can repeat to heal and release negative emotions. By repeating it several times, you progressively erase memories and improve your attitude. You gradually free yourself from guilt and resentment.

Step Number 5: Close the process with gratitude. Thank your subconscious and supraconscious mind. Consciously thank yourself for the participation, the communication, the work, the cleansing, and the release result received. Trust that your inner divinity will bring the best for you, especially if you continue to work with love and forgiveness in your heart, with a true feeling of gratitude and desire for change.

Repeat this process several times to facilitate better and better communication between the three aspects of the self in relation to the problem. Thus, each time you practice Hoʻoponopono to solve something or in relation to something, you will have more opportunities to reach all the subconscious information and cleanse your memories more deeply. You will become more aware of your memories, the inspiration, and the behaviors you need to change in your daily situations.

*** Recommendations for performing the Ho'oponopono exercise:**

This therapy is often essential. It is recommended to repeat it several times and constantly every day. For best results, you can follow the recommendations below:

1. Become aware of the problem, analyze it, and go deep into the results you wish to obtain with the exercise.

2. Inwardly declare that you will begin the process.

3. Relax before you start and take the time to do some energizing breathing.

4. Keep the dialogue with the three minds (conscious, subconscious and supraconscious) asking for cleansing.

5. Repeat the 4 phrases of the mantra: sorry, sorry, thank you, I love you.

6. Listen at all times to the inspiration that may arise in that moment of meditation.

7. Connect with a sense of commitment, love, forgiveness, and gratitude, creating a positive charge for the duration of the practice.

You may get distracted or have to attend to something going on around you. Relax, it happens and it's okay. Simply return to the situation and continue with the 4 phrases of the mantra (sorry, sorry, thank you, I love you). When you want to finish, thank the participation of the three minds (conscious, subconscious and supra conscious) and state that the practice is over for the moment.

CHAPTER IV: BIODESCODIFICACIÓN AND BIONEUROEMOTION AS ALTERNATIVE THERAPIES

Part One: Historical context, review of the beginnings of Biodescodification and Bioneuroemotion.

Howdy! I am glad you have reached this chapter of the book. In it, I will share with you a little of the historical and theoretical context of how Biodescodification and Bioneuroemotion were born. This brief review of the origins of both disciplines will allow us to better understand their evolution through the years and the achievements that have been reached from the studies related to the association, thoughts, and emotion, as well as the relationship that exists between the body and the mind.

These modern therapeutic disciplines currently promote the reordering of the psychic-emotional aspects so that, with it, we reach a better well-being and integral health. It is important to emphasize that the Biodescodification is not born from a single researcher, but it comes from numerous sources. Among the most prominent people who exerted influence on a lesser or greater degree in the origins of Biodescodification are the following:

- *Sigmund Freud (1856-1939): Austrian neurologist of Jewish origin, father of psychoanalysis and one of the greatest intellectual figures of the 20th century. His influence: "Words have magic and power".*

- *Carl Gustav Jung (1875-1961): Swiss psychiatrist, psychologist and essayist, key figure in the initial stage of psychoanalysis; later, founder of the school of analytical psychology, also called psychology of complexes and depth psychology. His influence: "He discovers the collective unconscious and leaves the phrase 'Illness is a cry for healing'".*

- *Milton Erickson (1901-1980): born in Nevada, United States, was an American physician and hypnotherapist, innovator, and pioneer in changing the techniques of hypnotism applied to psychotherapy. He is recognized as the grandfather of modern hypnosis and is said to be the best hypnotherapist who ever lived. His influence: "Father of conversational hypnosis and was one of the models that influenced the beginnings of NLP and other psychotherapies".*

*- **Ernest Lawrence Rossi** (1933): psychologist, psychoanalyst, psychotherapist and teacher and student of Milton Erickson. Explorer of "mind-body psychobiology and healing powers" on the neuroscientific and genetic basis. His influence: "Author of Dialogue with Genes and Ultradian Theory".*

*- **Ryke Geerd Hamer** (1953): disqualified German physician. Creator of the Germanic medicine. He is known as the original father who influenced the first origins of Biodescodification. His influence: "Creator of the New Germanic Medicine".*

*- **Louise Hay** (1926): American writer and speaker, considered one of the most representative figures of the new thought movement. Precursor of self-help books, known worldwide for her book "You can heal your life". Her influence: "Positive Self-Affirmations to Heal the Body and Mind", creator of the first facsimile of diseases and their emotional causes.*

*- **Dahlke Rudiger and Thorwald Dethlefsen** (1984): The former, Dahlke, a scholar of occultism and astrology applied to psychological diagnosis. During the 1970s he conducted several experiments with hypnosis and developed the therapy of healing reincarnation. The second, Dethlefsen, is known for his numerous books and articles on health issues. His work focused on psychosomatics, spiritual philosophy, nutrition, and esotericism. His influence: "Authors of the book Disease as a Path".*

*- **Salomon Sellam** (1955): Doctor of Medicine (1983) and graduate in psychosomatic medicine and relaxation therapy (1995). He devoted much of his time to the diffusion of the psychosomatic clinic, a discipline he founded in 2000 following numerous consultations and the training of mental and physical health professionals. His influence: "He was the driving force behind Dr. Hamer's transgenerational theory. He also had a great influence on psychosomatic medicine".*

*- **Claude Sabbah** (1947): based on the theory of Dr. Ryke Geerd Hamer, having studied directly with him, he founded Total Biology, taking Hamer's findings to a new therapeutic perspective. His influence: "He focuses on a global vision of the human being, his experiences and the solution to revert many ailments and diseases from the understanding and resolution of the original conflict programming of the same".*

*- **Marc Fréchet** (1945): developer of "memorized cellular biological cycles" as well as other hologram concepts applied to biology to achieve healing. His influence: "The biological program of a given disease may even stem from an unresolved conflict in the genealogy of the individual".*

*- **Christian Fléche** (1957): father of the biological decoding of diseases and founder of the French school of "Décodage Biologique". He tells us that the original biological decoding is a therapeutic and health approach based on the biological meaning or sense of the symptoms of disease. He assures us that decoding is a path towards understanding the disease and the mechanisms that allow healing the consciousness and, in this way, healing the body. His influence: "He first coined the name: original biological decoding. A form of accompaniment that made it possible to know the coding mechanism of diseases, whether physical, functional, organic, psychological, or behavioral".*

*- **Enric Corbera** (1954): graduate in psychology and industrial engineer. After dedicating more than twenty years to research and training in various disciplines, he promotes in a close and understandable way a holistic vision of well-being. He achieved that the "bio" (abbreviation that we will use to designate the methodologies of the Biodescodificación, as well as the Bioneuroemoción) was legally officialized in Cuba as a healing therapy and was subject of the faculty of medicine. His influence: "Dedicated to the study of the psychic-emotional causes behind diseases. Develops emotional healing and was the first to use the term Bioneuroemotion".*

In summary, we can affirm that, although there are several characters in history that contributed to the study and later emergence of Biodescodification and Bioneuroemotion, these two disciplines coincide in that they deny the biological origin of the diseases and assure that the cure passes through the resolution of our emotional conflicts. We can say then that the two most influential characters are the postulates of "**Ryke Geerd Hamer**, creator of the **Germanic New Medicine**", which was one of the currents that inspired what would later be called Biodescodification; and the postulates of Enric Corbera, creator of the Bioneuroemotion method that promulgates that the world we see reflects our internal frame of reference and that our perception is based on interpretations, not on facts.

*** Points to consider:**

Well, since we studied a little bit of history of the beginnings and evolution of where the terms and studies of Biodescodification and Bioneuroemotion were born, now we will analyze the most outstanding findings of the most outstanding pioneers of these great disciplines. Among one of the most influential as we have previously studied was Dr. Ryke Geerd Hamer.

Dr. Hamer received terrible news in August 1978: his 19-year-old son Dirk had been accidentally shot while hunting on a holiday trip in the Mediterranean. Three months later, his son Dirk died. Shortly after this, Dr. Hamer, who had been in good health all his life, discovered that he had developed testicular cancer. Suspicious of this coincidence in relation to his son's death, he began to do research into the personal histories of cancer patients to see if they had suffered any shock, stress, or trauma prior to their illness.

Eventually, after extensive research with thousands of patients, Dr. Hamer came to the conclusion that many psychosomatic illnesses often occur after having experienced a very intense and surprising shock. This led him to create his well-known and famous theory: "Hamer's 5 Laws". Theory that later led to the creation of "The German New Medicine".

Part Two: Evolution of Biodescodification:

Biodescodification continued to evolve through the years thanks to the contributions of Marc Fréchet, clinical psychologist who studied together with Claude Sabbah the theory of Dr. Hamer having both studied directly with him. They took Hamer's findings to a new therapeutic perspective and asked themselves: why do I resent what I resent? They discovered that this resentment was related to their history. They contributed important concepts, including the idea that the biological program of a given disease may even stem from an unresolved conflict in the genealogy of the individual.

The aforementioned Dr. Claude Sabbah, born in 1947 in Casablanca, also a physician (graduated from the universities of Marseille and Paris), oncologist specialized in sports emergencies, hyperbaric medicine, NLP psychotherapy based on the theory of Dr. Hamer and having studied directly with him, founded Total Biology, bringing Hamer's findings to a new therapeutic perspective that focuses on a global vision of the human being.

His experiences and the solution to reverse many ailments and diseases from the understanding of the resolution of the original conflict. Similarly, the aforementioned Dr. Salomon Sellam, also a disciple of Dr. Hamer, developed both the transgenerational theory and the rediscovery of the well-known "Gisant Syndrome". These different evolutionary processes allowed us to better understand the importance of transgenerational therapy in our lives.

According to his research, he found that the transgenerational transmission of the emotional memories we inherit from our ancestors and the emotional imprint we receive from our mother from before conception, during pregnancy, at birth and up to eight years of age is what sometimes generates hereditary diseases.

And finally, Dr. Enric Corbera, dedicated to the study of the psychic-emotional causes behind diseases. He develops emotional healing. Since, according to his theory, emotion is what gives meaning to our life. And that, for this reason, by finding the blocked emotion, Bioneuroemotion can be performed unblocking the causes that produce diseases or internal self-sabotage. Allowing practitioners spectacular improvements and a more holistic balance between thought and emotion, body, and mind. Bringing as a result a more balanced, healthy, and free of psychosomatic diseases.

Adopting the name of Bioneuroemotion in their therapies instead of Biodescodificación. Arguing that the latter was an evolution focused more on emotions.

Part Three: Differences Between Biodescodification and Bioneuroemotion

Both Biodescodification and Bioneuroemotion focus on investigating the relationship between emotions and the body. The Bioneuroemotion and the Biodescodification have as similarity that they are methods of consultation oriented to increase the physical and emotional well-being. Both methodologies use inquiry with the objective of identifying the origin of emotional conflicts and help to understand the relationship and the direct influence that exists between emotions and health.

Although they may seem similar, in reality they are very different methodologies both in their approach and in the techniques used and the results obtained. This is a natural evolution in coherence with the latest research and advances in various fields such as emotional management, neuroscience, psychoneuroimmunology, and current humanistic psychology trends.

*** What are the main differences?**

While Biodescodification associates a type of emotional conflict to each type of physical symptom, Bioneuroemotion avoids falling into determinisms. Unlike Biodescodification, Bioneuroemotion is based on the assumption that diseases are multifactorial. We know that each person is a world and that no two cases have the same history. For this reason, Bioneuroemotion takes much more into account the particularities of each person and has multiple tools that allow us to decipher the real root of the conflict.

On the other hand, Biodescodification is a proposal of alternative medicine that tries to find the metaphysical origin of the diseases or their emotional meaning in order to find from there a way to heal.

Through Biodescodification therapies, the therapist looks for new codes to be activated in the cells of the body so that health can be restored or function in a normal way and give a better quality of life to the person. This emotional therapy optimizes each one of the treatments that the patient receives, teaching the person to improve his/her concentration, to listen to the most intimate part of the organism, as well as to listen to the biology of his/her body and psychological health.

*** Points to consider:**

As we can appreciate, each methodology has something in common, while at the same time they have very noticeable differences between them. The important thing is that both methodologies have proven over time to be excellent therapeutic tools that are very valuable in improving people's health and personal well-being. Each has its advantages depending on the case, situation, and circumstance. Therefore, knowing and understanding the benefits they bring to our wellbeing make them unbeatable allies for health.

*** Other information of interest:**

Psychoneuroimmunology (PNI) is the science that deals with the relationship between thoughts, feelings, and actions. That is, it is the science that studies the interaction between the psychic processes, the nervous system (NS), the immune system (IS) and the endocrine system (ES) of the human body and the bodily processes that influence each other. Thanks to it, the relationship between the mind and the body with certain psychosomatic diseases, functional disorders and even psychic imbalances is becoming more and more evident.

Regarding the impact that our mind-body perceptions have on the state of the human being. Aldous Huxley teaches us that: "Experience is not what happens to a man, but what that man does with the experience that happens to him". To reinforce the above idea, we will quote a phrase from Marcus Aurelius that says: "If you feel distressed by any external thing, the pain is not due to the thing itself, but to your own estimation of it; so, you have the power to remove it at any time".

By way of recapitulation, the origins of Biodescodification gain strength thanks to the fusion between transgenerational therapy and many of the elements of other disciplines such as Germanic medicine. Disciplines and therapies that were gradually incorporated generated a new and recent methodology: the Bioneuroemotion promoted by Dr. Enric Corbera. The advances of scientific research in the last decades together with the most avant-garde of modern psychotherapy focused on the body-mind-thought-emotion processes. Both disciplines have shown better results in people than traditional orthodox treatments.

Part Four: Other Basic Concepts and Definitions

Biodescodification and Bioneuroemotion, as we have learned so far, could be defined as one of the most innovative and effective natural healing proposals to help the individual to recover the holistic balance, body-mind, thought-emotion. Bringing as a result a healthier and integrally balanced life.

Through these methodologies we learn to listen to what our body, mind, thoughts, and emotions want to tell us. Through the study of neurobiology and neurology (referring to thoughts and ideas, as well as physiological, biological, and emotional reactions that are produced by the individual) it has been proven that certain diseases manifest themselves through conditions, symptoms, discomfort, stress, psychic-emotional disorders, among others.

And both neurobiology and neurology act as a primary guide by which we can be guided to initiate a deep healing process of healing. Through certain effective procedures that are intended to eradicate the cause of the deep-seated internal self-sabotage that is generating the disease and thus begin the healing of the body and mind.

***How is Biodescodification carried out?**

The neurons in our body contain and record information. This information comes in each person, from genetic inheritance, from the life of each individual, from what he knows, feels, thinks and lives. Each neuron is coded and programmed with this information, which activates its functioning and causes our cells, tissues, and systems to behave in a certain way.

Biodescodification consists of activating new codes in the cells and creating new, more empowered neuronal patterns that allow these neurons to recover a healthier and more harmonious behavior.

***Why do we get sick?**

The perspective of the methodology applied in Biodescodification as well as in Bioneuroemotion tells us that illness is the consequence of our way of thinking, feeling, and acting before life situations. Our personal beliefs (mental maps or paradigms) originate codes in our cells or neuronal grooves, which cause the body to manifest either optimal health or generate diseases that are mostly psychosomatic.

In other words, if we have limiting thoughts, feelings, or ways of acting or ways of seeing life that are conditioned or not very conscious, it is possible that the disease will manifest itself more viably. However, it is also true that if our way of living is balanced and holistic, we will enjoy better well-being and integral health.

*** Objectives of Biodescodification.**

The objective of Biodescodification is to find the biological sense of the symptom so that the patient becomes aware of the answer that "the unconscious is giving as a biological solution" and in this way sees the healing process as a possible way. Clearly understanding of course that the disease is something external and that it has to do in most cases with our thoughts, emotions and behaviors. By becoming aware that these limiting actions carry within them a manifest disease.

The healing process is much faster, since when knowing the cause that produced the symptom, it is much easier to correct the disorder. In other words, the Biodescodification aims to lead the person who is ill to the following question: What is it that has led me to this health condition? Why does my biology express itself in this way? What does my body want to tell me and what should I revise in my life?

Part Five: Biodescodification Evolves to Bioneuroemotion.

It is important to emphasize that initially in the beginnings of these disciplines the Biodescodification was used as a method of biological origin of dual vision. Focused mainly on seeking physical health and complementing orthodox medical treatments to improve their effectiveness through the search for behavioral solutions and the search for physical and corporal health.

As therapies evolved and combined with other alternative psycho-therapeutic branches focused more on the mind-body, the focus of Biodescodification changed from the biological part to the neurological and emotional part. That is to say, it moved from focusing on the biological processes (symptom/illness) to focus on the neurological processes (thoughts, feelings/emotions and actions = response). This resulted in the emergence of the new term: Bioneuroemotion.

This new methodology is a way of living that seeks personal well-being in holistic balance between mind, thoughts, emotions, and actions. Today, Bio-neuroemotion covers all areas of the person and responds not only to physical problems but also to interpersonal and social difficulties. In short, Bioneuroemotion covers all situations that provoke psychic-emotional conflicts, seeking to expand consciousness in a more humanistic way, becoming one of the most effective healing tools.

With the emergence of Bioneuroemotion, the aim is to transcend unconscious individual, family, and cultural beliefs in order to achieve emotional freedom. Promoting the perspective that everything we live has to do with us and therefore with our well-being. Hence, we can stop being victims of a situation (manifest disease) and have the power to heal ourselves and transform any ailment by changing our perception in a more ecological condition, focused on a better lifestyle, healthier and balanced between our thoughts, emotions, and actions.

*** Bioneuroemotion as a means of alternative therapy.**

We are usually accustomed or rather conditioned to look for the solution to our health problems in a conscious place. That is, we try to fix the symptoms of diseases with a limited and self-sabotaging way of seeing reality through medicines, treatments or therapies that are a set of means of any kind (hygienic, pharmacological, surgical, medical, or physical) whose purpose is the cure or temporary relief of diseases.

However, to truly initiate a healthy alternative therapy process that offers us a true healing, regenerative, healing, and liberating response, it is proposed to focus beyond our conscious self-sabotaging limiting consciousness.

And to reach that unconscious part of ourselves that is often ignored, but that powerfully and drastically influences our well-being. In the power of the unconscious or subconscious mind is where we find amazing answers to what the body manifests. Becoming aware of our internal saboteur through what we feel, and think is the key to the methodology applied in Bioneuroemotion to recover the health of the body and the psychic-emotional well-being in an integral way.

Because when internal emotional self-sabotage occurs in the form of thoughts or feelings formed either by your beliefs, ideas, experiences, or opinions by channeling and channeling them to our own advantage, we can begin to work on these manifestations (diseases or symptoms) and heal or release them.

One of the fundamental principles of the applied Biodescodification and the conscious Bioneuroemotion as a means of alternative therapies is that the therapist accompanies the person who suffers some type of discomfort so that he/she can speak and freely express his/her hidden emotions, thoughts and feelings while becoming aware of that internal self-sabotage that does not allow him/her to identify with the problem. The solutions to health complications are found in what the patient may not be able to face or what has gone unnoticed or unimportant to him/her.

It is crucial to remember that many of these negative emotions are only the reflection of our thoughts and feelings together with the repetition of certain habits and mental conditioning that are the result of limiting patterns and programming. Situations that when presented consecutively and permanently communicate to us that there is something inadequate that we must improve or correct.

Part Six: Symbolic Meaning of Diseases: Problem, Probable Cause and New Mental Model.

As you go through the following list, see if you can find the correlation between the disease you have or the symptom you have suffered and the probable causes that have originated the condition. You will not only understand the biological origin of the discomfort, but you will also have a set of recommendations that will allow you to work on that manifest symptom through affirmations and the New Mental Model of biological coding.

Affirmations and mental model that allows us to release and recode those energetic charges that produce that event in the organism, reprogramming our mind cells and neuronal circuits, bringing as a result a remarkable improvement in your health and well-being. You can use this list when you have a physical problem and want to know the symbolic meaning that represents each disease. And thus, be able to work that energetic charge, release it and let flow the stagnant emotion that produced the ailment using the biological coding used in Biodescodification therapies as well as in Bioneuroemotion therapies to treat diseases from a more holistic therapeutic alternative that has given excellent results through the last decades.

To begin, look at the emotional cause and see if it applies to you. If not, ask yourself silently what the thoughts, feelings or actions that generated that particular problem might have been.

Repeat to yourself, "**I am willing to give up the mental model that has created this problem.**"

Repeat several times the New Mental Model that we propose.

And take it for granted that you are already in the healing process. Declare it, believe it, and declare healing and liberation in your life.

Every time you think about your current state, repeat the steps of the New Mental Model and act on that new belief.

Index of Diseases, Causes and Solution

- **Abdominals, spasms** ≥ emotion that produces it: fear.
   New Mental Model: I trust the process of life. I am safe.
   - **Miscarriage** ≥ emotion that produces it: fear.

New Mental Pattern: Divine protection is always at work in my life. I love and approve of myself. All is well.

- **Abscesses** ≥ fear of the future. Procrastination, not now; later.

New Mental Model: I allow my thoughts to be free and allow myself to take action now.

- **Accidents** ≥ inability to speak in self-defense, rebellion against authority, reliance on violence.

New Mental Model: I free myself from the mental model that originated this situation. I am at peace. I am worthy and valuable.

- **Acidity** ≥ fear. Suspicion. Doubt. Paralyzing fear.

New Mental Model: I breathe freely and fully. I am safe. I trust the process of life. I feel safe and move forward.

- **Acne** ≥ disapproval and lack of acceptance of self.

New Mental Model: I am a divine expression of life. I love and accept myself as I am now.

- **Addictions** ≥ escape from oneself. Fear. Someone who does not know how to love himself.

New Mental Model: Now I discover how valuable I am, and I decide to love and enjoy myself and life.

- **Adrenals** ≥ problems of defeatism. Someone who is no longer interested in themselves. Anxiety.

New Mental Model: I accept and love myself. By taking care of myself I am safe and secure.

- **Alcoholism** ≥ what's the point? Feeling of futility, guilt, and inadequacy. Self-rejection.

New Mental Model: I live in the here and now. Every moment is new. I dare to see my own value; I love and approve of myself as I am.

- **Allergies** ≥ ask yourself who you are allergic to. Denial of one's own power. Discomfort towards a close one.

New Mental Model: The world is safe and friendly. I am safe. I am at peace with life. I accept people with their faults and virtues.

- **Alzheimer's disease, disease of** ≥ desire to leave the planet. Inability to face life as it is.

New Mental Model: Everything happens in the proper spatiotemporal sequence. Divine right action happens in every moment and in every place.

- **Tonsillitis** ≥ fear. Repressed emotions. Stifled creativity.

New Mental Model: My good flows freely. Divine ideas are expressed through me. I am at peace with myself and my environment.

- **Amnesia** ≥ fear. Flight from life. Inability to defend oneself.

New Mental Model: Intelligence, courage and self-confidence never fail me. There is no risk in being alive. There is much to live for.

- **Blisters** ≥ resistance. Lack of emotional protection.

New Mental Model: I flow smoothly with life and with each new experience. All is well.

- **Anemia** ≥ "yes, but" attitude. Lack of joy. Fear of life. Feeling of not being good enough.

New Mental Model: I can safely feel joy in all areas of my life. I love life, I love to live and be happy.

- **Sickle cell disease** ≥ someone whose belief that they are "good for nothing" destroys their joy of life.

New Mental Model: this child lives and breathes the joy of living, and love nourishes me. God works miracles every day in my life.

- **Angina** ≥ intense belief that one is incapable of asserting oneself and asking for what one needs.

New Mental Model: I have the right to have my needs met. I am able to ask for what I want, easily and with love.

- **Distress** ≥ lack of confidence in the movement and process of life.

New Mental Model: I love myself; I approve of myself, and I trust the process of life. I am safe. I feel full confidence and security.

- **Ano** ≥ point of release. Waste disposal.

New Mental Model: I easily and comfortably release what I no longer need in life. I let go of what needs to go and release it with love.

- **Abscesses** ≥ anger in relation to that which one does not want to let go of.

New Mental Model: there is no danger in loosening up. Only what I no longer need leaves my body. Everything negative flows out of my life easily.

- **Itching** ≥ guilt about the past. Remorse.

New Mental Model: with love I forgive myself. I am free from my past.

- **Pain** ≥ guilt. Desire for punishment. "I'm no good for..."

New Mental Model: let bygones be bygones. I decide to love and approve myself in the present. I know I am capable; I know I can, and I will.

- **Hemorrhage** or **anorectal** ≥ anger and frustration.

New Mental Model: I trust the process of life. In my life there is nothing but right and good actions. And I thank life for that.

- **Anorexia** ≥ denial of one's own life. Much fear. Self-rejection. Self-hatred.

New Mental Model: by being myself I am safe. I am fine just as I am. I choose life, joy, and acceptance of myself.

- **Apathy** ≥ resistance to feeling. Dampening of the self. Fear.

New Mental Model: there is no danger in feeling. I open myself to life and I am willing to live it. I open myself to be more empathetic with people.

- **Appendicitis** ≥ fear. Fear of life. The flow of good is blocked.

New Mental Model: I am safe. I relax and let life flow joyfully. I am free, I feel safe, and I flow normally.

- **Excessive appetite** ≥ fear. Need for protection. Attitude of judging emotions.

New Mental Model: I am safe. There is no danger in feeling. My feelings are normal and acceptable. I love and want myself as I am.

- **Appetite**, **loss of** ≥ fear. Protection of self. Lack of confidence in life.

New Mental Model: I love myself; I approve of myself, and I am safe. Life is safe and joyful. I feel protection and security in everything I do.

- **Wrinkles** ≥ stem from depressive thoughts. Resentment with life.

New Mental Model: I express the joy of living and allow myself to fully enjoy every moment of the day. I rejuvenate and feel jovial.

- **Arteries** ≥ fear of the joy of living. Worry and anguish.

New Mental Model: I am filled with joy that flows through me with every heartbeat. My life flows naturally and I feel great.

- **Arteriosclerosis** ≥ resistance, tension. Rigidity and narrow-mindedness. Refusal to see the good.

New Mental Model: I open myself completely to life and joy, and I choose to see with love. I am flexible in creative and positive thinking.

- **Articulations** ≥ represent changes in life orientation and the ease or difficulty with which they are carried out.

New Mental Model: I flow easily with change. My life is guided by the divine, and I always move in the best direction.

- Arthritis ≥ feeling of being unloved. Criticism, resentment.

New Mental Model: I am love, I decide to love and approve myself. I see with love and approval all the good things I do.

- Finger arthritis ≥ desire to punish. Guilt. Someone who feels victimized.

New Mental Model: I see with love and understanding, and I elevate all my experiences to the light of love.

- Rheumatoid arthritis ≥ deep criticism of authority. Someone who feels very exploited.

New Mental Model: I am my own authority. I love and approve of myself. Life is good.

- Choking, attacks of ≥ fear. Distrust of the process of life.

New Mental Model: there is no danger in growing up. The world is a safe place. I am safe. I am confident and secure in what is to come.

- Asthma ≥ suffocating love. Inability to breathe alone. Choking sensation. Suppressed crying.

New Mental Model: there is no danger in me now taking charge of my own life. I choose to be free. I feel liberated and relaxed in every moment of my life.

- Asthma in infants ≥ fear of life. Someone who doesn't want to be here.

New Mental Model: this child is received with love and joy and is safe and well cared for. I love this baby; he is a wonderful being who brings joy to my life at every moment.

- Seizure (cardiac, apoplectic) ≥ hopelessness. Endurance. Rather die than change. Refusal of life.

New Mental Model: life is change, and I adapt easily to the new. I accept life, past, present, and future. I feel I have a zest for life, and I look forward to each new day to live it more intensely.

- Spleen ≥ miscellaneous obsessions.

New Mental Model: I love and approve of myself. I trust the process of life. I am safe. All is well and I am calmly going about my life.

- Mouth ≥ represents the incorporation of new ideas and nourishment.

New Mental Model: I nourish myself with love. I open myself to new ideas.

- Sores, in mouth ≥ festering words that lips withhold. Guilt.

New Mental Model: In my world of love, I only create joyful experiences. Everything I say and express is positive and full of good vibes.

- **Problems, from the mouth** ≥ rigid opinions. Closed mindedness. Inability to accept new ideas.

New Mental Model: I welcome new ideas and digest and assimilate them in a good way, with joy, love, and hope.

- **Arms** ≥ represent the ability to embrace life experiences.

New Mental Model: I receive and welcome my experiences with love and joy. I open myself to new experiences with love and gratitude.

- **Bronchitis** ≥ difficulties in the family environment. Arguments and shouting. Sometimes silence.

New Mental Model: I declare peace and harmony within myself and with my surroundings. All is well in my home and there is harmony in my family group.

- **Head**, **pains of** ≥ someone who invalidates himself. Self-criticism. Fear.

New Mental Model: I love and approve of myself. I see myself and everything I do with love. I am in harmony with my surroundings and environment. I love and accept myself as I am.

- **Hip** ≥ carries the body in perfect balance. The main thrust in the forward movement.

New Mental Model: every day I move forward with joy. I am in perfect balance with the universe, and I always move forward with joy.

- **Problems, hip** ≥ fear of making important decisions. No direction to move forward.

New Mental Model: I am in perfect balance. At any age, I move through life with joy and ease.

- **Cramping** ≥ tension, fear. To cling, to hold on to.

New Mental Model: I relax and let my mind be still. I feel safe, I let my thoughts free and flow freely.

- **Gallstones** ≥ bitterness. Cruel thoughts. Condemnation. Pride.

New Mental Model: I feel liberation from the past and gratitude for the experiences I have gone through. Life is sweet, beautiful, and pleasant. I am sweet, attentive and feel empathy for the people around me.

- **Calluses** ≥ hardening of concepts and ideas. Solidified fear.

New Mental Model: I feel safe in experiencing new ideas and attitudes. I open myself to receive all the good that the universe has prepared for me.

- **Baldness** ≥ fear. Tension. Attempt to control everything. Lack of confidence in the process of life.

New Mental Model: I am safe. I love and approve of myself as I am, I trust life and let everything flow freely.

- **Gray hair** ≥ stress. Nervous tension, overexertion.

New Mental Model: I am at peace with all aspects of my life. I am strong and capable. I take things in stride and relax. I feel calm and live in harmony with my surroundings and loved ones.

- **Cancer** ≥ deep wound. Resentment that creeps in. Someone who is eaten away by a deep pain or secret. Burden of hatred. Belief that everything is useless.

New Mental Model: I forgive with love and let go of all the past. I choose to carry my world with joy and happiness. I love and approve of myself. I feel love for myself and express it to others. My life is a little box of surprises that surprises me every day with good things that make me happy and grateful on a daily basis.

- **Candidiasis** ≥ feeling of being very scattered. Frustration and anger. Demands and distrust in relationships.

New Mental Model: I allow myself to be all that I can be, and I deserve the best in life. I love and appreciate myself, and I love and appreciate others.

- **Cara** ≥ represents what we show to the world.

New Mental Model: I am safe being who I am, and I express myself as I am. I am honest with myself and transparent. I show myself to others as I am. I like and empathize with the people around me.

- **Cataracts** ≥ inability to look ahead with joy. Bleak future.

New Mental Model: life is eternal and full of joy. I look forward with hope, my future is positive and full of opportunities.

- **Cellulite** ≥ someone stuck in childhood sufferings, clinging to the past. Difficulty in moving forward. Fear of choosing one's own direction.

New Mental Model: I forgive everyone, and I forgive myself. I forgive all past experience. I am free and let all past experience flow with joy and new hope.

- **Brain** ≥ represents the computer, the program of our beliefs, habits, and behaviors.

New Mental Model: I am the loving operator of my mind. I reprogram my mind with positive and empowered beliefs, habits, and behaviors.

- **Tumor** ≥ misinformation of beliefs. Obstinacy. Refusal to change old mental models.

New Mental Model: I can easily reprogram my mental computer. Everything in life is change; my mind is always positive. I adapt to change and open myself to new opportunities.

- **Sciatica** ≥ hypocrisy. Fear of money and the future.

New Mental Model: I go into my own good. My good is everywhere; I am safe and secure. I open myself to abundance and prosperity. I am a magnet to attract economic opportunities into my life.

- **Elbow** ≥ represents changes in direction and acceptance of new experiences.

New Mental Model: I flow easily with new experiences and changes of direction. I accept change and adapt to new opportunities that come my way.

- **Cholesterol** ≥ obstruction of the channels of joy. Fear of accepting joy.

New Mental Model: I decide to love life. The channels of my joy are open. I open myself to receive joy in my life and all that is good.

- **Colic** ≥ mental irritation, impatience, annoyance with the environment.

New Mental Model: my inner child responds to love, to thoughts of love and everything is at peace in my inner being.

- **Colitis** ≥ overly demanding parents. Fear of oppression and defeat. Great need for affection.

New Mental Model: I love, approve, and accept myself as I am. I create my own joy and choose to succeed in life.

- **Colon, mucus in the** ≥ accumulation of old confused thoughts clogging the elimination channel. Someone who lingers in the sticky mire of the past.

New Mental Model: I let go of the past and dissolve it. My thoughts are clear. I am in peace and joy with myself, I live in the present, in the here and now.

- **Spine** ≥ the flexible life support.

New Mental Model: life supports me and conspires in my favor. Everything that happens in my life is for the best and I receive it with joy and gratitude.

- **Spine, stooped** ≥ inability to flow with the support of life. Fear and attempt to cling to old ideas. Lack of faith in life. Lack of integrity. Someone who lacks the courage to follow his or her convictions.

New Mental Model: I free myself from all fears and trust the process of life. I know that life is good and positive for me. With love I stand up, straight and tall in the face of all circumstances that life presents to me.

- **Itching** ≥ unwelcome desires. Dissatisfaction. Remorse for leaving or turning away.

New Mental Model: I am at peace where I am. I accept my good, and I know that all my needs and all my desires will be fulfilled.

- **Conjunctivitis** ≥ anger and frustration at what one sees in life.

New Mental Model: I see with the eyes of love. There is a harmonious solution for all the things I do, I accept my life with love and joy, and I feel grateful for all the blessings I receive.

- **Heart** (see also blood) represents the center of love and security.

New Mental Model: my heart beats to the rhythm of love. I live my life at a calm, joyful, happy pace and in harmony with my life purpose.

- **Problems, of heart** ≥ old emotional problems. Hardening of the heart. Tension and stress.

New Mental Model: jubilation. Joy. Joy. I lovingly allow joy to flow through my mind, my body, and my experience. I close cycles of the past, let the present flow and free myself from all emotional energetic charges. I live my life in relaxation, inner peace, and harmony.

- **Attack on the heart** ≥ someone who, for money, position, does not live his life in a harmonious way, removes from his heart all joy and all joyfulness.

New Mental Model: I return joy to the center of my heart. To all I express my love. I attract love into my life. I love and receive love in abundance.

- **Neck** ≥ represents flexibility. The ability to see what is behind.

New Mental Model: I am at peace with life. I am flexible in all aspects of my existence. I have the ability to look at my past with joy, live in my present and prepare positively for my future.

- **Neck, problems of** ≥ refusal to see more than one aspect of an issue. Stubbornness, inflexibility.

New Mental Model: I easily see all aspects of a problem and find creative solutions. There are endless ways of doing and looking at things. I am grateful to have a variety of options and alternatives to get things done in my daily life.

- **Neck, stiffness of the** ≥ inflexible obstinacy.

New Mental Model: it is safe to see other points of view. I am able to see and accept other points of view different from my way of thinking, I am flexible, and I adapt to changes easily.

- **Fingers** ≥ represent the details of life.

New Mental Model: I am at peace with the details of life.

- **Thumb** ≥ **thumb** represents intellect and concern.

New Mental Model: my mind is at peace.

- **Index finger** ≥ represents the inner self and fear.

New Mental Model: I am safe and secure.

- **Middle finger** ≥ represents anger and sexuality.

New Mental Model: I am comfortable with my sexuality.

- **Ring finger** ≥ represents unions and mourning.

New Mental Model: I peacefully give love.

- **Little finger** ≥ represents family and falsehood.

New Mental Model: I am myself with my family, I am myself before life and with all the people who know me.

- **Depression** ≥ grief. Fear of inspiring life. Someone who feels unworthy of living fully.

New Mental Model: I have the capacity to inspire the fullness of life, and with love I live it fully.

- **Fainting** ≥ fear that cannot be faced. Loss of consciousness.

New Mental Model: there is no danger in being myself. I express who I am. I make myself known to the world and to people as I am.

- **Diabetes** ≥ nostalgia for what may have been. Great need to control. Deep sadness. No trace of sweetness.

New Mental Model: this moment is full of joy. I choose to experience the sweetness of everyday life. I am happy, joyful, and content.

- **Diarrhea** ≥ fear. Rejection. Flight.

New Mental Model: my intake, assimilation and elimination are in order. I am "at peace with myself...". I feel secure and confident.

- **Teeth** ≥ represent decisions. Problems of old indecision. Inability to break down ideas to analyze and decide.

New Mental Model: I make my decisions based on the principles of truth, and rest easy knowing that I live my life in harmony and inner peace.

- **Muscular dystrophy** ≥ extreme fear. Frantic desire to control everything and everyone. Deep need to feel secure. Loss of faith and confidence. No danger in being alive or being myself.

New Mental Model: it's okay to be the way I am, and I have confidence in myself. I am an extraordinary, kind, and gentle person.

- **Continuous pain** ≥ longing for love. Longing to be embraced.

New Mental Model: I love, accept, and approve of myself as I am. I am capable of loving and being loved, I am worthy of love and receiving love.

- **Pain** ≥ guilt. Guilt always seeks punishment.

New Mental Model: with love I free myself from the past. They are free and so am I. All is well in my heart. I live in finite harmony with the universe, I feel liberated from the bonds of the past.

- **Eczema** ≥ intense antagonism. Mental eruptions.

New Mental Model: harmony, peace, love, and joy surround me and dwell within me. I am safe, secure, and happy with my life.

- **Edema** ≥ what or who do you not want to part with?

New Mental Model: I willingly renounce the past. It is safe to free myself from it, and now I am free. What has to go with love I let go of. I open myself to receive new experiences and free myself from the past.

- **Gums, problems of** ≥ inability to maintain decisions. Indifference to life.

New Mental Model: I am a decisive person, and I support myself with love. I have the ability to make my own decisions.

- **Bleeding gums** ≥ lack of joy in life decisions.

New Mental Model: in my life there is always the right action. I am at peace and in harmony with myself. I am happy and content.

- **Chronic diseases** ≥ refusal to change. Fear of the future. Lack of sense of security.

New Mental Model: I am ready to change and grow. I am creating a new, secure, and better future for myself. I am grateful to life.

- **Numbness** ≥ withholding of love and consideration.

New Mental Model: I respond to the love in everyone. I am considerate and loving. I share my feelings and love with everyone.

- **Epilepsy** ≥ feeling of persecution and intense struggle. Rejection of life. Self-imposed violence.

New Mental Model: I choose to see life as eternal and joyful. I am eternal and joyful; I am at peace and happy with myself.

- **Equilibrium, loss of** ≥ scattered, unfocused thinking.

New Mental Model: I focus on safety and accept the goodness in my life. All is well in my life and around everything I do.

- **Belching** ≥ fear. Someone who swallows life too quickly.

New Mental Model: there is time and space for everything I need to do. I am at peace and live in harmony every moment of my life.

- **Eruptions** ≥ irritation due to delays. Childish way of attracting attention.

New Mental Model: I love, accept, and approve of myself as I am. I am at peace with the process of life. I am joyful and happy every day.

- **Chills** ≥ mental contraction, withdrawal, and withdrawal. Desire to withdraw and be left alone.

New Mental Model: I am safe and secure at all times. Love surrounds me and protects me. All is well and safe around me.

- **Scleroderma** ≥ feeling of helplessness and insecurity. Someone who feels irritated and threatened by others.

New Mental Model: I am divinely protected; I am safe at all times. Everything I do is good and brings me love, which I accept with pleasure and joy. I feel protection and security in my life.

- **Multiple sclerosis** ≥ mental rigidity, hardness of heart, iron will, inflexibility. Fear.

New Mental Model: by choosing to love and joyful thoughts I create a kind and joyful world for myself. I feel free, happy, and safe.

- **Scoliosis** ≥ see backs, loaded back represents life support.

New Mental Model: I know that life is good and always supports me.

- **Back,** ≥ upper back **problems**, lack of emotional support. Feeling of not being loved. Withholding of love.

New Mental Model: I love, accept, and approve of myself as I am. Life supports me and loves me. I give love and receive abundant love.

- **Back** middle part ≥ guilt. Someone stuck in the past, whom he sees as a burden.

New Mental Model: I let go of the past. I am free to move forward with love in my heart. I move forward and trust that all will be well.

- **Low back** ≥ fear of running out of money. Lack of financial support.

New Mental Model: I trust the process of life, which always takes care of everything I need. I am financially and economically well.

- **Back, burdened with** ≥ someone who carries the weight of life. Helplessness and hopelessness.

New Mental Model: I stand tall and free. I love and approve of myself. My life gets better day by day. And I free myself from all the burdens of the past.

- **Pimples** ≥ someone who feels dirty and unloved.

New Mental Model: I love, accept, and approve of myself as I am. I love and am worthy of love. I feel comfortable with myself.

- **Sterility** ≥ fear and resistance to the process of life or lack of need to have the experience of motherhood (or fatherhood).

New Mental Model: I trust the process of life. I am always in the right place doing the right thing at the right time. I love and approve of myself. I am worthy of loving and worthy of receiving love.

- **Stomach** ≥ contains food. Digests ideas.

New Mental Model: I easily digest life. I easily assimilate all life processes and flow freely with ease.

- **Constipation** ≥ refusal to give up old ideas. Someone who is stuck in the past. Sometimes pettiness.

New Mental Model: as I let go of the past, the new, the fresh and the vital come into me. I allow life to flow through me. I free myself from the past and flow freely into my future.

- **Fatigue** ≥ endurance, boredom, Lack of love for what is being done.

New Mental Model: I am full of energy and enthusiasm for life.

- **Uterine fibroids** and **cysts** ≥ someone who cultivates resentment toward her partner A blow to the female self.

New Mental Model: I renounce the mental model that provoked this experience I only create good, love and loving harmony in my life.

- **Cystic fibrosis** ≥ firm belief that life will not work for one.

New Mental Model: life loves me and I "love" it, I choose to receive it fully and freely my future. I open myself to all that is good and flow freely.

- **Hay fever** ≥ emotional congestion. Fear of the calendar. Someone who feels persecuted. Guilt.

New Mental Model: I am one with the totality of life. I am safe at all times. I let my emotions flow freely and lovingly.

- **Fevers** ≥ scorching cholera.

New Mental Model: I am a calm and serene expression of peace and love. I am at peace and in harmony with myself and others.

- **Fistula** ≥ fear. Blockage in the release process.

New Mental Model: I am safe. I trust the process of life because it belongs to me. I flow in life with freedom, safety, and love.

- **Phlebitis** ≥ anger and frustration. Someone who blames others for the limitation and lack of joy in their life.

New Mental Model: joy flows freely within me, and I am at peace with life. I forgive with love and live in joy with everyone.

- **Fluids**, **retention of** ≥ what are you afraid of losing?

New Mental Model: I joyfully let flow and free myself every day.

- **Boils** ≥ boiling cholera.

New Mental Model: I express love and joy, and I am at peace every day.

- **Frigidity** ≥ fear. Denial of pleasure. Belief that sexuality is bad. Insensitive partner.

New Mental Model: I am glad to be a woman. It is good to enjoy my own body and live my sexuality freely without taboos or fears.

- **Gangrene** ≥ mental morbidity. Poisonous thoughts suffocate joy.

New Mental Pattern: I choose harmonious thoughts and let joy flow through me. I am happy and alive, joyful every moment of the day.

- **Throat** ≥ channel of expression and creativity.

New Mental Model: I open my heart and sing the joys of life.

- **Gases, pain due to** ≥ contracture. Fear. Undigested ideas.

New Mental Model: I relax and let life flow freely through me. I love and approve of myself. I digest ideas with ease.

- **Gastritis** ≥ prolonged uncertainty. Fatalistic feeling.

New Mental Model: I love, accept, and approve of myself as I am. I am happy with myself and live in harmony with my environment.

- **Genitalia** ≥ represent the male and female principles.

New Mental Model: I love, accept, and approve of myself as I am. I am a person worthy of love and worthy of receiving love, affection, and passion.

- **Glands** ≥ represent supply stations. They are the initiating activity.

New Mental Model: in my world I am the creative power.

- **Glandular**, **problems** ≥ poor distribution of mobilization ideas, I have the ideas and activity I need, I march forward Gordura.

New Mental Model: my ideas are valuable and contribute to my life and my social environment Divine love protects me I am safe and secure.

- **Gout** ≥ need for dominance, impatience anger.

New Mental Model: I am safe, secure, at peace with myself and others I am a patient, tolerant, loving, calm person.

- **Influenza** ≥ reaction to negative mass beliefs. Fear. Faith in statistics.

New Mental Model: I am beyond the beliefs or the group calendar, and free of all congestion and influence.

- **Hemorrhages** ≥ jubilation escapes. Anger. But where?

New Mental Model: I am the joy of life that expresses and receives in a perfect rhythm. I live in love and harmony with everyone around me.

- **Hemorrhoids** ≥ fear of deadlines. Anger with the past. Fear of slacking off. Feeling of being overloaded.

New Mental Model: I free myself from everything that is not love. There is time and place for everything I want to do. My life flows with freedom, harmony and my time is enough to do everything that makes me happy.

- **Hepatitis** ≥ resistance to change. Fear, anger, hatred. The liver is the seat of anger and rage.

New Mental Model: my mind is free and clear. I renounce the past and move on to the new. All is well in my life.

- **Hernia** ≥ rupture of relations. Tension, burdens. Incorrect creative expression.

New Mental Model: my mind is soft and harmonious. I love and approve of myself. I am free to be me. I live tension-free and stress-free.

- **Herniated disc** ≥ feeling of receiving no life support. Indecisiveness.

New Mental Model: life supports all my thoughts; therefore, I love and approve of myself, and all is well in my life.

- **Herpes** ≥ belief in sexual guilt and need for punishment. Public shame. Faith in an unforgiving god. Rejection of genitalia.

New Mental Model: my concept of God supports me. I am normal and natural. I am happy with my sexuality and my body. I am worthy of love.

- **Liver** ≥ seat of anger and primitive emotions.

New Mental Model: love, peace and joy are what I profess.

- **Swelling** ≥ stuck, pelleted, and painful ideas.

New Mental Model: my ideas flow freely and easily; I move freely between them. My life flows freely and so do my ideas.

- **Hyperglycemia** ≥ see diabetes.

- **Hyperthyroidism** ≥ disappointment at not being able to do what one wants. Someone who always tries to satisfy others and almost never himself.

New Mental Model: I put my power back in the right place. I make my own decisions and I am happy to choose what is best for my life.

- **Hyperventilation** ≥ fear, resistance to change, distrust of life process.

New Mental Model: I am safe anywhere in the universe. I love and trust the process of life.

- **Hypoglycemia** ≥ someone overwhelmed by the burdens of life, who continually wonders: what good is it?

New Mental Model: I choose to make my life simple, easy, and joyful. I feel liberated and I know that the decisions I make are good ones.

- **Shoulders** ≥ are made to carry joys, not burdens.

New Mental Model: I feel unburdened and joyful to live.

- **Bones** ≥ represent the structure of the universe.

New Mental Model: I am well-structured and balanced.

- **Bones, problems of** ≥ deformities, strains, mental pressures. Muscles that cannot stretch. Loss of mental mobility.

New Mental Model: I fully inspire life. I relax I trust the flow of life process. I move with flexible ease.

- **Fractures** ≥ rebellion against authority.

New Mental Model: I respect authority and am conscious of my actions. I avoid offending and disrespecting others.

- **Inflammation of the ileum** ≥ fear and worry about "not serving".

New Mental Model: I love and approve of myself. I am doing my best to serve and help others. I am perfect. I am at peace.

- **Impotence** ≥ sexual pressure, tension, and guilt. Social beliefs. Resentment against a previous partner. Fear.

New Mental Model: I allow the full power of my sexual principle to operate easily and joyfully. My sex life is healthy and beautiful.

- **Incontinence** ≥ letting go. Feeling of loss of emotional control. Lack of self-nourishment.

New Mental Model: by nourishing myself I take care of my health and well-being. I nurture those around me with love and kindness. I am tender and loving.

- **Indigestion** ≥ visceral fear, terror, anguish.

New Mental Model: I digest and assimilate joyfully and peacefully every new experience. I feel security, peace, and tranquility. I assimilate my experiences gladly. I move forward and flow naturally.

- **Infection** ≥ irritation, anger, annoyance.

New Mental Model: I choose to be in peace and harmony. I live my life with tranquility, joy, and love. I feel happy every moment of the day.

- **Urinary tract infections** ≥ someone who feels irritated usually by a lover or other individual of the opposite sex. Someone who blames others.

New Mental Model: I renounce the mental model that created this condition. I set out to change for the better. I love myself; I accept myself; I approve of myself as I am.

- **Inflammation** ≥ fear Someone who is out of his or her mind Inflamed thinking.

New Mental Model: my thinking is peaceful, serene, centered.

- **Insomnia** ≥ fear, lack of confidence, process, life, guilt.

New Mental Pattern: with love I say goodbye day I let myself go sleep peacefully second tomorrow everything will resolve itself My life flows everyday peace serenity.

- **Intestines** ≥ represents release of waste.

New Mental Model: it is easy for me to let go and let love flow all emotions limiting thoughts.

- **Laryngitis** ≥ someone is so angry, can't speak. Fear of asserting oneself. Resentment of authority.

New Mental Model: I am free to ask for it. It is safe to express myself freely. I am at peace with others.

- **Leukemia** ≥ brutal death, inspiration. Someone continually says all useless.

New Mental Model: beyond past limitations in, freedom, present moment. It is certain who I am.

- **Leucorrhea** ≥ belief woman has no power opposite sex. Anger, partner.

New Mental Model: I create all experiences. I am power. I enjoy being a woman, I am free to love and be loved.

- **Lymph problems** ≥ warning there is refocusing mind essential life love joy.

New Mental Model: center totally, love, joy, being alive I flow freely, my life, peace of mind.

- **Lupus** ≥ resignation. It is considered better to assert oneself. Anger, punishment.

New Mental Model: I assert myself, freely, easily. I claim power. I love myself; I approve of myself; I am safe and free.

- **Bruises** ≥ life's little bumps can lead to self-punishment.

New Mental Model: I love and care for myself. I am kind and tender with myself. All is well in my life, and I flow with freedom and love.

- **Bad breath** ≥ may be caused by ideas of anger and revenge, supported by experiences.

New Mental Model: with love I let go of the past. I decide to express my love freely, I am happy and live my life joyfully.

- **Jaw problems** ≥ can be caused by anger, resentment, and desire for revenge.

New Mental Model: I love, approve, and accept myself as I am. I am safe and feel secure in showing love and receiving love.

- **Hands** ≥ hold and handle, grasp and loosen, caress and pinch. They are all ways of coping with experiences.

New Mental Model: I choose to handle all my experiences easily, with love and joy. I am flexible and flow freely every day.

- **Travel sickness** ≥ can be caused by fear, especially of death and lack of control.

New Mental Model: I am totally safe in the universe and at peace everywhere. I trust in life and divine protection.

- **Meningitis** ≥ can be caused by major family discord, an atmosphere of anger and fear, inner turmoil, and lack of support.

New Mental Model: I create peace in my mind, my body, and my world. All is well around me. I am safe and I am loved.

- **Problems, of menopause** ≥ can be caused by fear of no longer being loved and growing old, self-rejection and thoughts such as "I am no good".

New Mental Model: I feel balanced and serene in all cycle changes, I bless my body with love, tenderness, and acceptance.

- **Menstrual problems** ≥ may be caused by rejection of one's femininity, guilt, fear, and belief that the genitals are sinful or unclean.

New Mental Model: I accept my full power as a woman and accept as normal and natural all the processes of my body. I love, accept, and approve of myself as I am.

- **Migraines** ≥ may be caused by dislike of letting go, resistance to the flow of life, or sexual fears (usually masturbation can alleviate them).

New Mental Model: I relax in the flow of life and let it easily provide me with everything I need.

- **Myopia** ≥ may be caused by fear of the future or distrust of what is to come.

New Mental Model: I trust the process of life. I am safe.

- **Mononucleosis** ≥ may affect someone with a mental pattern that leads to devaluing life or aggravating others; someone with a lot of internal criticism or habit of playing "isn't it terrible?".

New Mental Model: I am one with the totality of life; I see myself with others and I like what I see; I rejoice in being alive, healthy, and happy.

- **Motion sickness** ≥ may be caused by fear of being out of control.

New Mental Model: I always control my thoughts; I am safe; I love, accept, and approve of myself as I am.

- **Problems with** ≥ **wisdom teeth** can affect someone who does not give themselves mental space to create a firm foundation.

New Mental Model: I open my consciousness to the expansion of life; there is abundant space for me to grow and change.

- **Women's problems** ≥ may be caused by self-denial or rejection of the feminine principle.

New Mental Model: I rejoice in my femininity; I like being a woman; I love my body; I accept it as it is.

- **Doll** ≥ represents movement and looseness.

New Mental Model: I handle all my experiences easily, with love and prudence. I flow with ease in all aspects of my life.

- **Birth,** ≥ karmic **defects.** You chose to come this way. We choose our parents.

New Mental Model: every experience is perfect for our growth process. I am at peace and in harmony where I am.

- **Buttocks** ≥ represent power. Loose buttocks, lack of power.

New Mental Model: I use my power wisely. I am strong. I feel secure. All is well in all aspects of my life.

- **Narcolepsy** ≥ inability to cope. Extreme fear. Someone who wants to get away from it all, and not be here.

New Mental Model: I trust divine wisdom to protect and guide me always. I am safe, secure and feel confident.

- **Nose** ≥ represents recognition of oneself.

New Mental Model: I recognize my own intuitive capacity.

- **Nasal, hemorrhage** ≥ need for recognition. Feeling of not being recognized and going unnoticed. Someone crying out for love.

New Mental Model: I love, accept, and approve of myself as I am. I recognize my own value. I am perfect and live in divine harmony.

- **Nausea** ≥ fear. Rejection of an idea or experience.

New Mental Model: I am safe. I trust that the process of life brings me nothing but good. Every experience is good.

- **Nephritis** ≥ overreaction to disappointment and failure.

New Mental Model: in my life there is only right action. I let go of the old and welcome everything new. All is well.

- **Nerves** ≥ represent information. They are information receptors.

New Mental Model: I communicate easily and happily with everyone.

- **Nervous, crisis** ≥ self-centered. Communication channel blockages.

New Mental Model: I open my heart to create only harmonious communications. I am safe, I am well and secure.

- **Nervousness** ≥ fear, anguish, pugnacity, precipitation. Distrust of the process of life.

New Mental Model: I go on an endless journey through eternity, and I have plenty of time. I communicate with my heart. All is well in my life.

- **Pneumonia** ≥ someone desperate, tired of life. Emotional wounds that are not allowed to heal.

New Mental Pattern: I freely absorb divine ideas, filled with the inspiration and intelligence of life. I free myself from the wounds of the past. I forgive and free myself from the past and flow freely every day.

- **Neuralgia** ≥ feeling of guilt. Self-punishment. Distress about communication.

New Mental Model: I forgive, love, and approve of myself as I am. I communicate with love. It is easy for me to express myself to others.

- **Nodules** ≥ selfish resentment and frustration over career.

New Mental Model: I let go of the pattern of delay and let success be mine. I flow freely and let myself be carried by the good things in life.

- **Ears** ≥ represent the ability to hear.

New Mental Model: I hear with love.

- **Eyes** ≥ represent the ability to see clearly past, present, and future.

New Mental Model: I see my present and future with love and joy.

- **Eyes, problems** ≥ someone who doesn't like what they see in their life.

New Mental Model: I am creating a life that I love to look at. I see my present with joy and love to see the good things in life.

- **Astigmatism** ≥ I disturb. Fear of actually seeing oneself.

New Mental Model: I am ready to see my inner beauty and magnificence. I am an excellent human being.

- **Cataracts** ≥ inability to look forward with jubilation. Bleak future.

New Mental Model: life is eternal and full of joy.

- **Reddened** ≥ anger and frustration. Someone who does not want to see.

New Mental Model: I renounce the need to be right. I am at peace. I love, accept, and approve of myself as I am.

- **Convergent strabismus** ≥ someone who does not want to see what is outside. Contradictory purposes.

New Mental Model: it is safe to look ahead. I am at peace.

- **Divergent strabismus** ≥ fear of looking at the present, the here and now.

New Mental Model: I love and approve of myself in the here and now.

- **Glaucoma** ≥ steely refusal to forgive. Pressure from very old wounds. Someone overwhelmed by it all.

New Mental Model: I see with love and tenderness. I love my life, forgive my past and release the emotions that limit my potential.

- **Myopia** ≥ fear of the future.

New Mental Model: I accept divine guidance and am always safe.

- **Presbyopia** ≥ fear of the present.

New Mental Model: I see that I am safe here and now.

- **Body odor** ≥ fear. Dislike of self. Fear of others.

New Mental Model: I love, accept, and approve of myself as I am.

- **Ovaries** ≥ represent points of creativity.

New Mental Model: my creative process is balanced.

- **Pancreas** ≥ represents the sweetness of life.

New Mental Model: my life is sweet.

- **Pancreatitis** ≥ rejection. Frustration and anger because life seems to have lost its sweetness.

New Mental Model: I love, accept, and approve of myself as I am. I am creating sweetness and joy in my life.

- **Paralysis** ≥ fear, terror. Flight from a situation or a person. Resistance.

New Mental Model: I am one with the totality of life. I am safe, and I feel totally adequate for any situation.

- **Parkinson's disease, disease of** ≥ fear and intense desire to control everything and everyone.

New Mental Model: I relax in the certainty that there is no danger. Life belongs to me, and I trust its process.

- **Breasts, problems with** ≥ lumps, cysts, hypersensitivity. Exaggeration of maternal attitude. Overprotection. Despotic attitudes. Withdrawal of food.

New Mental Model: I am free to be myself and leave others free to be who they are.

- **Peptic, ulcer** ≥ fear. Someone who thinks he or she is "no good...". Anxiety to please.

New Mental Model: I love, accept, and approve of myself as I am. I am at peace with myself. I am perfect.

- **Weight, excess** ≥ fear, need for protection. Flight from feelings. Insecurity, rejection of self.

New Mental Model: I create my own security; I accept my feelings. I love, accept, and approve of myself as I am.

- **Athlete's foot** ≥ frustration at not being accepted. Inability to advance easily.

New Mental Model: I love, accept, and approve of myself as I am. I allow myself to move forward. There is no danger in moving.

- **Skin** ≥ protects our individuality and is a sensory organ.

New Mental Model: I feel safe being myself.

- **Legs** ≥ carry us forward in life.

New Mental Model: life belongs to me.

- **Legs, problems of the** ≥ upper part: someone who clings to old childhood traumas.

New Mental Model: they acted to the best of their ability with the understanding, awareness, and knowledge they had. I set them free.

- **Legs, problems of the** ≥ lower part: fear of the future. Refusal to move.

New Mental Model: I move forward with confidence and joy, knowing that all is well in my future.

- **Feet** ≥ represents our understanding of ourselves, of life, of others.

New Mental Model: my understanding is clear, and I am willing to change with the times. I am safe.

- **Pyorrhea** ≥ anger at the inability to make decisions. Indecisive people.

New Mental Model: I approve of myself, and my decisions are perfect for me.

- **Pituitary**, **gland** ≥ represents the control center.

New Mental Model: my mind and body are in perfect balance, and I control my thoughts and emotions.

- **High blood pressure** ≥ old, unresolved emotional problem.

New Mental Model: I joyfully let go of the past. I am at peace.

- **Prostate** ≥ represents the male principle.

New Mental Model: I accept my masculinity with joy.

- **Psoriasis** ≥ fear of being hurt. Dampening of the senses and the self. Refusal to accept responsibility for one's feelings.

New Mental Model: I open myself to the joys of life. I deserve and accept the best of it. I love and approve of myself as I am.

- **Pubic**, **bone** ≥ represents genital protection.

New Mental Model: my sexuality is safe.

- **Lung** problems of ≥ the ability to inspire life.

New Mental Model: I am in perfect balance, I inspire life.

- **Burning** ≥ anger. Someone who burns with fury.

New Mental Model: in myself and in my environment, I only create peace and joy. I deserve to feel good.

- **Cysts** ≥ someone replaying an old painful movie and cultivating grievances. False growths.

New Mental Model: the movies in my mind are beautiful because that is how I choose them. I love myself; I accept myself and I love myself as I am.

- **Rage** ≥ anger. Belief that violence is the answer.

New Mental Model: I am surrounded by love and full of peace and harmony.

- **Rectum** ≥ see anus.

- **Cold** ≥ too many things happening together. Confusion and mental disorder. Small grievances. Belief that "every winter, three colds."

New Mental Model: I let my mind relax and feel at peace. Clarity and harmony surround me, and love is within me.

- **Breathing** ≥ represents the ability to breathe in life.

New Mental Model: I love life.

- **Rheumatism** ≥ feeling of being a victim. Lack of love. Chronic bitterness, resentment.

New Mental Model: I create my own experiences. Love and approval from myself and others make my experiences better and better.

- **Rigidity** ≥ rigid thinking.

New Mental Model: I feel confident enough to be mentally flexible.

- **Kidney, problems of** ≥ criticism, disappointment, failure. Embarrassment. Someone who reacts like a child.

New Mental Model: divine action always operates in my life. The result of every experience is good. It is sure to grow every day.

- **Knee** ≥ represents pride and self.

New Mental Model: I am flexible and fluid.

- **Snoring** ≥ stubborn refusal to abandon old mental models.

New Mental Model: I renounce everything that is not love and joy. From the past I move towards the new, fresh, and vital, flowing with freedom.

- **Blood** ≥ represents joy flowing freely through the body.

New Mental Model: I am the joy of living that is expressed and received.

- **Blood problems** ≥ lack of joy. Ideas do not circulate.

New Mental Model: new and joyful ideas circulate freely within me.

- **Clots** ≥ obstruct the flow of joy.

New Mental Model: I flow and awaken a new life within me.

- **Scabies** ≥ infected thought. Someone who allows "getting under their skin".

New Mental Model: I am the living, loving and joyful expression of life. I am master of myself.

- **Cranial sinuses, problems of the** ≥ irritation with someone very close.

New Mental Model: at all times, peace and harmony are in me and surround me. All is well.

- **AIDS** ≥ self-denial. Sexual guilt. Strong belief that one is "no good..."

New Mental Model: I am a magnificent and divine expression of life. I rejoice in my sexuality. I rejoice in all that I am. I love myself.

- **Syphilis** ≥ see venereal, diseases.

- **Premenstrual syndrome** ≥ someone who lets confusion reign and gives power to external influences. Rejection of female processes.

New Mental Model: I take charge of my mind and my life. I am a powerful woman. Every part of my body functions perfectly. I love myself.

- **Deafness** ≥ rejection, obstinacy, isolation. What is it that I don't want to hear "don't bother me".

New Mental Pattern: I hear the voice of the divine and rejoice in all that I am able to hear. I am one with wholeness.

- **Stuttering** ≥ insecurity. Lack of self-expression. Someone who is not allowed to cry.

New Mental Model: I am free to speak in my own defense. I am confident in my ability to express myself. I only communicate with love.

- **Had** ≥ someone convinced of being an impure and helpless victim in the face of other people's overt attitudes.

New Mental Model: Others only reflect the feelings I have for myself. I love and approve of all that I am.

- **Testes** ≥ the male principle, masculinity.

New Mental Model: It is completely safe to be a man.

- **Thyroid** ≥ humiliation. "I never get to do what I want, when will my turn come?".

New Mental Model: I transcend old limitations and allow myself to express myself freely and creatively.

- **Ankle** ≥ represents mobility and direction.

New Mental Model: I move forward easily in life.

- **Kinks** ≥ anger and resistance. Not wanting to move in a certain direction in life.

New Mental Model: I trust that the process of life is working for my good I am at peace and happy with myself.

- **Coronary thrombosis** ≥ feeling of loneliness and fear. "I'm no good...I don't do enough. I'll never make it."

New Mental Model: I am one with life. The universe fully supports me. All is well in my world and around me.

- **Tumors** ≥ someone who nurtures old wounds and generates remorse.

New Mental Model: with love I free myself from the past and attend to the new. All is well in my life.

- **Ulcers** ≥ fear. Someone who believes he is of no use... What is it that eats away at him?

New Mental Model: I love, accept, and approve of myself as I am. I feel at peace. All is well.

- **Urticaria** ≥ small hidden fears. Grains of sand become mountains.

New Mental Model: I bring peace to the last corner of my life.

- **Uterus** ≥ represents the home of creativity.

New Mental Model: my body is my home.

- **Nails** ≥ represent protection.

New Mental Model: I feel safe and protected.

- **Nail biting** ≥ frustration. Someone who eats himself. Resentment with a parent.

New Mental Model: It is safe to grow. I live with ease and joy.

- **Ingrown toenails** ≥ concern and guilt about one's own right to move forward.

New Mental Model: it is my divine right to choose my direction in life. I am safe. I am free and I flow freely.

- **Vaginitis** ≥ anger with partner. Sexual guilt. Self-punishment.

New Mental Model: others reflect the love and approval I feel for myself. I rejoice in my sexuality.

- **Bladder, problems of** ≥ distress. Someone clinging to old ideas. Fear of loosening up. Someone who feels irritated.

New Mental Pattern: I easily let go of the old and welcome the new into my life. I am safe and let my past flow freely with love.

- **Varicose veins** ≥ someone in a situation you dislike. Discouragement. Feeling of overwork and responsibilities.

New Mental Model: I am right, and I live in joy. I love life and flow freely.

- **Venereal, diseases** ≥ sexual guilt. Need for punishment. Belief that genitals are dirty or sinful. Abuse of others.

New Mental Model: With love and joy I accept my sexuality and its expression I only accept thoughts that support me and make me feel good I love, accept, and approve of myself as I am.

- **Small warts** ≥ expressions of hatred Conviction of ugliness.

New Mental Model: I am the full expression of love and the beauty of life.

- **Vertigo** ≥ flight of thoughts, dispersion Refusal to look.

New Mental Model: I am deeply centered and at peace with life It is completely safe to feel alive and joyful.

- **Vitiligo** ≥ not belonging Feeling of being completely out of it all and not being of the group.

New Mental Model: I am at the very center of life and totally connected to love.

- **Vulva** ≥ represents vulnerability.

New Mental Model: In the infinitude of life, where I am, everything is perfect, complete, and whole.

CHAPTER IV: EMOTIONAL RELEASE TECHNIQUE (EFT - TAPPING) - BALANCING AND RELEASING THE ENERGY CHANNELS OF THE HUMAN BODY

Part One: Historical Context and Overview of the Beginnings of the Emotional Freedom Technique (EFT - Tapping)

To begin this interesting chapter, I want to share a brief summary of what the Emotional Freedom Technique (EFT) is. It is a form of psychotherapy based on several theories of alternative medicine, including acupuncture, acupressure, acupressure, neuro-linguistic programming, energy medicine and thought field therapy (TFT). This procedure is a very effective self-help and emotional healing therapeutic tool for healing ourselves and freeing ourselves from self-sabotage. These are internal battles that are waged within our mind and body at every moment and are personified by that black wolf we learned about in the first chapter of the book.

Emotional Freedom Technique (EFT) works with our vital points or meridians, allowing us to channel our energy flow or Chi. This allows us to balance our energy channels and take control of our inner warrior or white wolf in the struggle to free ourselves from our inner emotional self-sabotage. And this is my intention for you. So, without further ado, let's continue.

"The cause of all negative emotions is an imbalance in the body's energy system." This phrase, in a nutshell, is the reason for the high success rate of the Emotional Freedom Technique or EFT. Every time you have a limiting thought or self-sabotaging memory of a past traumatic event, the normal flow of energy or Chi is interrupted.

That emotion *(self-destructive feeling or black wolf)* remains blocking your energetic system; and that is mostly experienced externally through physical pain, psychosomatic disorders, or a flurry of negative emotions.

In other words, internal emotional self-sabotage, or black wolf *(fear, hatred, anger, resentment, sadness, pain, loneliness, etc.)* are altered states of consciousness that cause knots and disorders in your body's energy system. When the energetic channels or meridians are tangled or misaligned, they produce within you an internal emotional battle that limits your movements, abilities, attitudes, thoughts, and emotions. These blockages or energetic knots produce all kinds of unwanted and unpleasant sensations, situations and emotions that affect both your mind and your body *(psyche-soma)*, producing alterations and even psychosomatic illnesses.

Thus, if you remove the blockage or energetic knots - not the thought or memory that produced it, but the stagnant energy - you automatically rebalance the normal energetic flow of the body. Consequently, it results in "freeing" your inner warrior or white wolf, allowing physical pain, psychosomatic disorders, and all bursts of negative emotions to fade away.

In other words, by simply applying the emotional release technique or EFT and tapping on some of the vital points or specific meridian points on your body, while at the same time repeating specific phrases to yourself, your energetic channels are released. Your vital energy or Chi flows freely again throughout your body allowing you to dissipate unpleasant and unwanted feelings by "releasing" your inner warrior or white wolf. This allows you to holistically balance both your mind and body *(psyche-soma)*, thus eliminating any existing psychosomatic illnesses.

According to Gary Craig, the technique of emotional release is a paradigm shift in the world of psychotherapy. Since EFT - Tapping is not part of the conventional techniques of alternative therapies, it is recommended to have an open and willing mind when practicing it. By correctly working EFT through tapping on our energetic channels, our body's energy is restored again and flows freely, allowing us to feel good once more. Completely freeing us from internal emotional self-sabotage. And that, my friend, is the end result that the Emotional Freedom Technique or EFT gives us.

*** What are the beginnings of the Emotional Freedom Technique (EFT)?**

In the 1970s, **psychologist Dr. Roger Callahan** combined elements of quantum theory, kinesiology, and acupuncture to begin healing patients with phobias and stress disorders. He used a system of different combinations of tactile and kinesthetic stimuli to stimulate different points by tapping on specific meridian points to heal different problems. This highly effective therapy was called "**Thought Field Therapy (TCP)**".

American psychotherapist Gary Craig, by then a Stanford engineer who studied with Dr. Callahan, extended the concept of thought field therapy (TFT) by devising a set of vital points or meridians more conducive to tapping, which he realized were easier to learn and remember.

He called his system "**Emotional Freedom Technique** or (**EFT**)". Since its conception, EFT - Tapping has gained worldwide acceptance and recognition with more and more practitioners, professional therapists and many other specialists around the world practicing the Emotional Freedom Technique (**EFT - Tapping**) as an alternative health therapy. Now more licensed emotional healers are also using EFT - Tapping as part of their repertoire. However, the basic technique has been made available to everyone yes, the same technique you will learn in this book.

*** What is the Emotional Freedom Technique (EFT)?**

Emotional Freedom Technique, or **EFT** for short, means "Emotional Freedom **Technique**". The Emotional Freedom Technique is part of a new category of procedures and protocols that are also known worldwide as "**energy therapies**" or "**therapies for the liberation of energy channels**". This methodology was created and developed by the renowned American psychotherapist Gary Craig.

The Emotional Freedom Technique is a short procedure that can be easily learned and applied to obtain a positive and transcendental dynamic change in our lives. EFT is based on the premise that the cause of all negative emotions is a disruption of the body's energetic flow. Tapping (an Anglo-Saxon term for a series of rhythmic "acupressure" taps used in EFT procedures) is a combination of very simple short phrases spoken out loud along with tactile stimulation of specific energy points in the body that restores the normal flow of energy channels.

Such stimulation of these energy points dislodges, disperses, and releases unwanted energy that has been blocked and allows our body's natural energy to re-establish itself and flow normally back into our system.

Today the technique of emotional release or EFT is part of the so-called "**techniques of advanced psychology**" alternative methods based on the belief that the mind and body are interconnected with each other and for this reason should be treated in a holistic and holistic synergistic way (as happens in traditional Chinese medicine).

Recall that the Emotional Freedom Technique or EFT is based on the premise that the cause of all emotional imbalance is an interruption of free flow in the body's energy system.

The Emotional Freedom Technique or EFT - Tapping works with the mind and the body in a double way. The physical intervention of the procedure is done through light physical contact "small touches or taps" *(kinesthetic touch)* that are executed in the meridians *(those vital points of the body where a greater amount of energy or Chi "used and known mostly in traditional Chinese acupuncture")*. While the psychological intervention is achieved by being consciously focused on the issue we want to treat through a "combination of very simple short phrases that are decreed out loud".

The "physical stimulation or intervention" *(kinesthetic contact)* being mentally focused on the problem we have "motivation of purpose" or psychological intervention *(verbal decree)* in 90% of the occasions manages to reestablish the free energetic flow and "release" that stagnant emotion. It should be noted that the memories of that particular event are still there, but the emotional charge that had been created and had been stuck in our body is released. This produces the release of the emotion and allows the normal energetic flow in the meridian points of the body to flow again, thus reestablishing the natural order of our energetic system.

Generally, one to three sessions of EFT - Tapping is enough to address simple discomforts that have not been ingrained in us for a long time, such as a heated argument, embarrassment after an embarrassing event, fear of a specific circumstance, small phobias, or traumas. And between seven to nine sessions of EFT - Tapping to address more serious or old socio-emotional wounds and to confront psychopathological problems that have been deriving in other new traumas or psychosomatic disorders.

   * **Who can use the emotional release technique?**

EFT - Tapping is beneficial for both men and women and can be used for infants, children, youth, adults, and the elderly. We can use it on ourselves *(self-tapping)* or on our family friends, known associates, patient clients and coachees.

Making the emotional release technique an excellent alternative to free ourselves from self-sabotage that are nothing more than internal battles that are waged within our mind at every moment always personified by that black wolf. In other words, the Emotional Freedom Technique (EFT) by working with our vital points or meridians allows us to channel our energy flow or Chi allowing us to balance our energy channels and take control of our inner warrior or white wolf in the struggle to free ourselves from our internal emotional self-sabotage.

The Emotional Freedom Technique or EFT - Tapping can be considered as a simple but effective procedure. It is an elegant, dynamic, and effective therapeutic process to release our energy channels and let the free flow of Chi energy flow again through the points or meridians of our body.

EFT - Tapping by combining psychology, quantum theory, acupuncture principles and other energetic processes from Asian cultures can be used to manage problems in almost any area of our lives, physical, emotional, mental, and spiritual. It can also be used to restore our relationships (family, couple, or work), harmonize with our finances, our surroundings or environment, with our dreams, goals, and objectives, it can also be used to connect with our sexual field and much more.

Part Two: How does the emotional release technique work?

EFT uses elements of acupuncture, but without using traditional needles. So tapping is referred to by many as acupressure *(kinesthetic contact with the fingertips or fingertips)* which serves to stimulate the meridians *(meridians are the energy channels or vital points through which energy or Chi flows).*

If you work on these specific points located on the skin that are very sensitive to touch, this contact positively influences the inside of our body. With this what we achieve is to allow the vital energy or "Chi" to flow freely again and "release" the stagnant emotion. The technique of emotional release or EFT - Tapping has a great advantage compared to other alternative therapies. The reason is that once learned and internalized the technique is very easy to use even unconsciously and anywhere without anyone around you noticing.

How do we learn to swim: by watching or by swimming, which would you rather have me talk to you about how to learn to swim or let you learn by getting in the water and letting you swim on your own?

In this short lesson I am going to share with you an allegorical example to transmit a very powerful teaching. My purpose at this point is to make you understand in a figurative way how you can learn the technique of emotional release in a very simple and easy way so that anyone can understand it and apply it to their own life. To start applying EFT - Tapping is a process in which you yourself must have the desire to do it and take action to make it happen and have the expected results in your own life.

Imagine that! It's like wanting to learn how to swim, but you only have the theory you acquired after reading a great book on swimming written by one of the best athletes in the world. Do you think just reading would make you a great swimmer? No, it wouldn't, would it? Reading is only part of what you need to do to achieve your purpose, right? The real challenge begins when you dive into the sea for the first time and start applying the knowledge you have read and learned in that extraordinary book. Now I ask you, do you think that just jumping into the pool for the first time is enough to make you a great athlete? No, isn't it? No, because that was just part of your training process to begin to develop the skills of an excellent swimmer. With continued practice is what will ultimately allow you to become what you set out to become. My invitation is that as you read this book you will jump into the water and practice what you are learning, and you will have step by step results on your way to personal excellence.

Interesting reflection, isn't it? Let me share another example, **how would you learn more about some fruit by eating it or by being told about it?** *For example, let's imagine I talk to you about a delicious and tasty apple, how would you learn more by letting me eat an apple or by letting me do both? As you may have already realized from this example, it is obvious that you would learn more about apples if you tried them yourself, even if you only ate a very small piece, than if I spent the next ten years telling you about them, right?*

In other words, my dear reader I could talk and teach you a lot about Emotional Freedom Technique or EFT - Tapping throughout this extraordinary book you are reading, but only until you experience it for yourself will you have a real idea of what these techniques can do for you.

Remember that in order to learn how to swim and know more about an apple what you have to do after reading is to put into action what you have learned. Of course, I would be happy to help you improve and correct the text you have provided.

To learn to swim, once you know the theory, you must dive into the water and practice to become the swimming athlete you want to be. Similarly, to learn more about an apple, you must taste it for yourself: feel its taste, texture, and shape; see its color and smell its aroma. Only then will that information become part of your unconscious records and you will be able to incorporate the information from the apple into your conscious mind. This will allow you to learn from your own experience more about it. The same happens with the technique of emotional release or EFT (tapping).

Now we come to the practical part, where we will learn how to use this technique which is very simple and practical once we know the steps to follow and comply with some essential principles. I will show you where are located each of the vital points of the basic and advanced recipe where you should do the "tapping" (kinesthetic contact with the fingertips to stimulate the meridians in each of the vital points). You can use either the right or left side of the body to tap and stimulate the energy channels; you can even change direction in the middle of a sequence or combine meridians if you feel you must. Remember that EFT (tapping) has an intuitive part.

The American psychotherapist **Gary Craig**, creator, and developer of EFT, recommends using your dominant hand for tapping *(the hand you use for writing)*. Therefore, if you are right-handed, it is usual to tap on the left side of your body; and if you are left-handed, on the right side. See how simple?

Before I continue, let me define a term we have talked about before: **"TAPPING"**. Tapping is an Anglo-Saxon term used to refer to a series of rhythmic tapping *(also known as "finger tapping")* used in EFT procedures. These taps are performed on each of the vital points or meridians indicated, gently but firmly and steadily.

Between five and nine touches for each marked point, although it is not necessary to count.

In short, EFT (tapping) combines very simple short phrases spoken aloud (purposeful motivation or psychological intervention) along with tactile stimulation of specific energy points on the body (physical stimulation or intervention), restoring the normal flow of energy channels.", "Stimulation of these energy points dislodges, disperses and releases unwanted energy that has become blocked. This allows our body's natural energy or Chi to re-establish and return to normal flow in our body's meridian system.

Basic Recipe or Basic Points:

Here I present the vital points, meridians or energy channels used in tapping. For a better understanding of the technique of emotional release, look closely at each of the graphics in the appendix that illustrate and represent "**the basic points of the EFT Basic Recipe - Tapping**".

- **Crown vital point (Co):**

This meridian point is sometimes also part of the basic recipe. **Crown**: upper part of the body: the crown or top of the head. This point is abbreviated as **Co**, for **Crown**.

Organ: corresponds to the bladder meridian. *Effect: releases fear and inhibition and enables courage.*

- **Third Eye Point** (**TO**): "*additional point of the advanced recipe*".

This point is located between the eyebrows, in the center of the forehead, in the area known as the "**Third Eye**" or the "**Ajna** or **Sixth Chakra**". This point is abbreviated as **TO**, for **Third Eye**. Organ: corresponds to the small intestine meridian. Effect: promotes mental clarity and intuition. And it belongs to the advanced recipe, which we will discuss in more depth later.

- **Vital points of the face "Ce, Lo, Bo, Bn and Bl".**

Beginning of the eyebrow: just where the eyebrow begins, where the bone behind the eyebrow meets the nose bone. This point is abbreviated as **Ce,** after the initial of eyebrow.

Side of the eye: would be where the eyebrow ends, at the rounded bone, at the outer edge that protects the eye laterally. That is, the bone on the side, which marks the corner of the eye. This point is abbreviated as **Lo,** for side of the eye.

Under the eye: over the bone just below the eye, in a vertical line with the pupil if you look straight ahead. That is, the bone in vertical line with the pupil, below the eye, over the cheek bone. This point is abbreviated as **Bo,** for under the eye.

Under the nose: just in the area between the nose and the upper lip. That is, in the small wavy u-shaped area in the center between the nose and the upper lip. This point is abbreviated as **Bn,** for under the nose.

Under the lips: just below the mouth, between the lower lip and the chin. That is; under the mouth, exactly under the lower lip and over the chin, between the center of both, where the beginning of the chin is marked. This point is abbreviated as **Bl,** for under the lips.

✓ Vital Points Crown "Co" and Face "Ce, Lo, Bo, Bn and Bl".

The abbreviations for these vital points, basic points, meridians, or energy channels in the above image are summarized in the same order in which they are presented above.

Co = center of crown

TO = center of the forehead "**Third Eye**", "**Ajna** or **Sixth Chakra**".

Ce = beginning of eyebrow

Lo = side of the eye

Bo = under the eye

Bn = under the nose

Bl = under the lips

- **Clavicle Vital Point (Cl)**

Clavicle point: this point is located at the beginning of the angle formed by the junction where the clavicle and the sternum begin. That is to say; it is the point of intersection where the sternum *(chest bone)*, the beginning of the clavicle and the first rib meet. This point is abbreviated as **Cl,** for **clavicle** *"although it does not lie exactly on it".*

- **Vital Points Under the Arm (Bb)**

Underarm: point located on the side of the body just below the armpit, at about the same height as the nipple in a horizontal line *(for men)* or halfway between the bra straps *(for women)*. In other words, this point is approximately 7 to 10 centimeters or about 4 fingers below the armpit. This point is abbreviated as **Bb,** for under the arm.

- **Vital Points, Collarbone and Under Arm "Cl, Bb".**

The abbreviations for these vital points, basic points, meridians, or energy channels in this image above are summarized in the same order in which they are presented above.

Cl = clavicle = basic recipe

Bb = under the arm = basic recipe

Advanced Recipe or Advanced Points:

Here I present the vital points, meridians or energy channels used in tapping. For a better understanding of this technique of emotional release, look closely at each of the graphics that illustrate and represent the advanced points in addition to the basic recipe of EFT- Tapping.

- **Third Eye Point (TO)**: *"additional point of the advanced recipe".*

This previously mentioned point is located between the eyebrows, in the center of the forehead, in the area known as the "**Third Eye**" or the "**Ajna or Sixth Chakra**". This point is abbreviated as **TO**, for **Third Eye**. Organ: corresponds to the small intestine meridian. Effect: promotes mental clarity and intuition.

*[This particular point **Third Eye (TO)** belongs to the Asian advanced recipe. At present, it is only used in some schools. For the purpose of this book. The point is considered important, so we mention it, and recommend its use].*

Note of interest: Buddhists consider the **third eye** as the "**eye of consciousness**". It is the sixth chakra, called **Ajna**. Representing the **Color: Violet** or **Indigo. Element: Light. Unlocks: Intuition.**

- **Sore Spot or Pain Zone (Ps - Zd) ORIGINAL ADVANCED RECIPE.**

The painful area is the point located on the sides of the chest where you would wear a button or badge *(showy or decorative ornament)*. To locate it just press gently with your fingertips until you locate an area on one side of the chest in the form of a small indentation or depression that is annoying and a little more painful to the touch than the others. That is to say; to locate the sensitive points what you should do is:

1.- place your index finger on the indentation between the clavicles.
2.- stretch your thumb and the rest of your fingers as much as possible.
3.- the sensitive point is the one located approximately at the end of the thumb and ring finger (ring).

If you do not feel pain or have the sensation of touching a weaker tender point, then feel around until you find that point that is more sensitive *(it feels that way because it is a lymphatic drainage point and is usually sensitive to touch; nothing will happen if you rub it, but avoid rubbing it too hard so as not to hurt yourself)*.

- **Advanced Vital Points Under the Breast or Under the Nipple (Bp - Bt). ORIGINAL ADVANCED RECIPE.**

This meridian point is sometimes part of the advanced recipe.
Under the Chest: this point would be located just below the pectoral muscles, in a vertical line with the ribs *(for men)* or where the breast ends for women, above the ribs *(for women)*. That is; it is located at the ribs, about 3 to 5 centimeters below the rib in men, and at the base of the chest for women, where the skin of the breast meets the chest wall. This point is abbreviated as **Bp,** for under the breast, or also as **Bt,** for under the nipple.
Note of interest: *This vital point is sometimes uncomfortable for women to locate. For this reason, there are therapists who eliminate it, however, it is very effective.*

- **Thymus point or Heart Chakra (TC):** *"additional point of the advanced recipe".*

Located in the center of the chest, slightly to the left, in the area of the "**Heart Chakra** or **Anahata**". This point is abbreviated as **TC**, for the "**Thymus**" gland and the Heart Chakra. **Organ**: corresponds to the pericardial meridian and the Thymus gland. **Effect**: promotes love, compassion, and emotional harmony; in turn, activates the immune system and cellular immunity.

*[This particular point **Timo or Heart Chakra (TC)** belongs to the Asian advanced recipe. At present, it is only used in some schools. For the purpose of this book. The point is considered important, so we mention it, and recommend its use].*

Note of interest: Buddhists consider the **Heart Point as the** "**Karmic Heart** or **Divine Flame of God**". It is the **fourth chakra**, called **Anahata**. Representing the **Color***: Green*. **Element***: Air*. **Unlocks**: *The capacity to love others and to open ourselves to life.*

- **Manipura Point** (MP): *"additional point of the advanced recipe".*

This point is located in the solar plexus area, just above the navel, in the area known as the "**Solar Plexus Chakra** or **Manipura**". This point is abbreviated as **MP**, for **Manipura**. **Organ**: corresponds to the meridian of the stomach and pancreas. **Effect**: strengthens self-esteem, personal power, and digestion.

*[This particular point **Manipura Point (MP)** belongs to the Asian advanced recipe. At present, it is only used in some schools. For the purpose of this book. The point is considered important, so we mention it, and recommend its use].*

Note of interest: Buddhists consider the **Manipura Point** as the "**Rising Sun**". It is the **Third Chakra**, called **Manipura**. Representing the **Color***: Yellow*. **Element***: Fire*. **Unlocks**: *Confidence and personal empowerment.*

Svadhisthana (SV) point: *"additional point of the advanced recipe".*

This point is located in the lower abdomen, approximately two fingers below the navel, in the area known as the "**Sacral Chakra** or **Svadhisthana**". This point is abbreviated as **SV**, for **Svadhisthana**. **Organ**: corresponds to the meridian of the kidneys and sex glands. **Effect**: stimulates creativity, pleasure, and sexual energy.

*[This particular **Svadhisthana (SV)** point belongs to the advanced Asian recipe. At present, it is only used in some schools. For the purpose of this book. The point is considered important, so we mention it, and recommend its use].*

Note of interest: Buddhists consider the **Sacral Point** as the "**Vessel of the Self**". It is the **Second Chakra**, called **Svadhisthana**. It represents the **Color**: *Orange*. Element: Water. Unlocks: *Sensuality and emotional connection.*

✓ **Vital Points Pain Point or Painful Zone "Ps or Zd, Bp or Pt" and Chakra Meridian Points "TO, TC, MP and SV".**

Vital Points Chest "Ps or Zd, Bp or Pt" ORIGINAL ADVANCED RECIPE

The abbreviations for these vital points, advanced points, meridians, or energy channels are summarized in the same order in which they are presented.

Point of interest: It is important to note that the meridian points used in EFT practice go downward (from top to bottom) through the body. This means that each tapping point is below the previous one. This allows you to memorize them in an instant in a very simple way when executed correctly. For this reason, I invite you to do some tapping through the vital points, basic points, meridians or energetic channels and you will see how you will learn them and remember them easily forever.

The abbreviations for these vital points, basic points, meridians, or energy channels are summarized in the same order in which they are presented.

TO = center of the forehead "**Third Eye**", "**Ajna** or **Sixth Chakra**".

Ps - Zd = tender point or painful area = advanced prescription.

TC = center of the chest "**Thymus-Heart**", "**Anahata** or **Fourth Chakra**".

Bp - Pt = under the breast "or" under the nipple = advanced prescription.

MP = above the navel "**Solar Plexus**", "**Manipura** or **Third Chakra**".

SV = below the navel "**Lower Abdomen**", "**Svadhisthana** or **Second Chakra**".

Vital Points of the Hand:

Vital Points of the Hand "Dp, Di, Dc, Dm; Gm, Pk and Mñ".

The energy points or meridians of the middle index thumb and little finger are located laterally in line with the base of the nail.

- **Points of the fingers of the hands:**

Thumb finger: this point is located on the underside of the nail at the outer base of the nail of your thumb in the direction facing the chest. That is, on the lower edge of the finger pointed in line with the base of the nail at the outer edge of the thumb farthest from the other fingers. This point is abbreviated as **Pu,** for thumb, or **Dp,** for thumb.

Index finger: this point is located on the underside of the nail at the outer base of the nail of your index finger (on the side closest to the thumb). That is, at the height of the base of the nail. This point is abbreviated as **Di,** for index finger.

Middle or **middle finger**: this point is located at the bottom of the nail at the height of the outer base of the nail of your middle or middle finger (on the side closest to the thumb). That is, at the height of the base of the nail. This point is abbreviated as **Dm,** or **Dmc,** for middle finger.

Little finger: this point is located on the underside of the nail at the outer base of the nail of your little finger (on the side closest to the thumb). That is, at the height of the base of the nail. This point is abbreviated as **Me,** or **Dme,** for little finger.

- **Point Gammas (PG):**

This point is located just before the knuckles of the little finger and ring finger in line with the central point between these two.

Gamma point: also known as "**gamma 9-range procedure (Gamut)**" which is located right at the crease at the top of the hand between the beginning of the little finger and the ring finger (ring) below the knuckles. In other words, the gamma point is the meridian point that is on the back of the hands, 1 centimeter below the center point between the knuckles at the base of the little finger and the ring finger. This point is abbreviated as **Pg,** for gamma point.

- **Karate Strike Point or Friendship Point:**

This point is located at the edge of the hand, at the point you would use to give a karate chop with the instep of it *(hence its name).* Or friendship point, because when we cordially extend our hand to a person by squeezing both hands we make a connection with this vital point, that is where we connect with others *(hence its name)*.

Karate point: is the point that is located on the lateral side of the hand in the intermediate point between the wrist and the birth of the little finger. That is to say; Karate point is located on the lower edge of the hand, in the fleshy middle between the wrist and the base of the little finger. This point is abbreviated as **Pk,** for karate point, or **Pa,** for friendship point.

- **Wrist point (Mñ or Mu):**

This point is located at the wrist, in the flexible and mobile part of the hand that allows its movement. Specifically, it is located on the lateral edge of the wrist, in the fleshy area between the wrist and the base of the little finger. You can easily identify it as the point where a watch or bracelet is placed on the wrist. This point is of great importance in EFT Tapping, and is abbreviated as Mñ, or Mu, for wrist.

It is important to note that EFT Tapping uses these vital points on the hand, including the wrist point, as part of the energy meridian stimulation technique to release emotional blockages and promote emotional and physical balance.

*** Point of Interest:**

The wrist point, within the context of EFT - Tapping, is used to stimulate the meridian called "**heart meridian**". By stimulating this point, we seek to release emotional blockages and promote emotional and physical balance related to the heart and emotions.

The heart meridian, according to traditional Chinese medicine, is associated with the physical organ of the heart and also with emotions and emotional well-being. By working on this point of the wrist, we seek to harmonize and balance the energy of the heart, releasing tensions and promoting a sense of calm and emotional well-being.

It is important to note that in the context of EFT - Tapping, the interpretation of the meridians and their relationship to the organs is symbolic and is based on the principles of traditional Chinese medicine. The effectiveness of EFT - Tapping is not limited to direct physical effects on the organs but focuses on energetic balancing and releasing emotional blockages.

- **Vital Points Hand "Dp, Di, Dm, or Dc, Me, or Dme" - "Gm, Pk and Mñ".**

The abbreviations for these vital points, basic points, meridians, or energetic channels above are summarized in the same order as presented above.

Dp = thumb.

Di = index finger.

Dm or Dc = middle "or" middle finger.

Me or Dme = little finger.

Pg = range.

Pk or Pa = karate "or" friendship.

Mñ or **Mu** = Wrist Point.

*** Points to consider.**

As we have learned so far, there are 21 vital points or at least these are the most known and used in tapping. For a better understanding of this technique of emotional release, look closely at each of the graphics that illustrate and represent the basic recipe along with additional advanced points of EFT-Tapping.

The abbreviations for these 21 vital points, basic points, meridians, or energy channels are summarized in the same order as presented above.

It is important to learn and memorize correctly all the vital points, basic points, meridians, or energetic channels. For this reason, take your time to locate each one of them, you will know that you are in the correct position because you will "feel" that this point is different from the others.

- **Vital Points Crown "Co" and Face "Ce, Lo, Bo, Bn, Bl".**

Co = center of crown

TO = center of the forehead "**Third Eye**", "**Ajna** or **Sixth Chakra**".

Ce = beginning of eyebrow

Lo = side of the eye

Bo = under the eye

Bn = under the nose

Bl = under the lips

- **Vital Points Basic Recipe - Chest "Cl, Bb".**

Cl = clavicle = basic recipe
Bb = under the arm = basic recipe

- **The Advanced Vital Points Sore Spot or Pain Zone and Under the Chest or Under the Nipple (Ps - Zd) (Bp - Bt) and the Chakra meridians: Thymus - Heart, Above the Navel and Below the Navel (TC, MP, SV).**

Ps - Zd = tender point or painful area = advanced prescription.
TC = center of the chest "**Thymus-Heart**", "**Anahata** or **Fourth Chakra**".
Bp - Pt = under the breast "or" under the nipple = advanced prescription.

MP = above the navel "**Solar Plexus**", "**Manipura** or **Third Chakra**".
SV = below the navel "**Lower Abdomen**", "**Svadhisthana** or **Second Chakra**".

- **Vital Points Hand "Dp, Di, Dm or Dc, Me or Dme" - "Gm, Pk and Mñ or Mu" - "Gm, Pk and Mñ or Mu".**

Dp = thumb
Di = index finger
Dm or Dc = middle "or" middle finger
Me or Dme = little finger
Pg = range
Pk Pa= karate "o" friendship
Mñ or **Mu** = Wrist Point.

To continue we can reaffirm that any energetic blockage in our meridian system can be properly released with this "**emotional release technique**" by applying **EFT- Tapping on the** following vital points of the basic and advanced recipe:

 * **Positive effects of the "Emotional Freedom Technique" applying EFT-Tapping.**

- Eliminates stress, anxiety, fears, phobias, insecurities, apathy, and depression.

- Release the emotions of anger, anger, resentment, guilt, sadness, loneliness, and grief.

- It helps us overcome frustration and internal self-sabotage.

- It allows us to begin a process to control and overcome addictions, such as: food, tobacco, alcohol, pornography, etc.

- It allows us to control the effects of obsessive-compulsive disorder.

- It allows us to reduce and relieve physical pain in general, such as: migraines, insomnia, fibromyalgia, tension, and muscular pain.

- It helps us to focus on what we want, allowing us to improve our learning capacity, academic performance, professional performance, sports performance, among others.

- It allows us to release emotional patterns that keep us anchored in scarcity and frustration.

Part Three: Basic Recipe of the EFT Processes Practical Exercises to Execute Tapping Points

In this book, as well as in the therapeutic sessions, face-to-face lectures and in the audio and video versions *(webinars and podcasts)* a modified version of the **"basic"** and **"advanced" EFT - Tapping technique** is used.

Next, I will explain in detail the basic and advanced steps in a series of practical exercises. But before doing so, I will share with you some preliminary concepts that are of vital importance to understand and correctly apply this technique of emotional release or EFT - Tapping.

"Problem recognition, preparation, intensity meter, reminder phrase, among others."

Once learned the basic and advanced recipe, these two recipes become our best ally throughout life in the practice of EFT - Tapping. The technique of emotional release can be applied for a large number of almost unlimited physical, mental, emotional, spiritual, psychological and psychosomatic problems, as it provides real and effective relief for most of them, allowing us to fade the physical-emotional pain, trauma or psychosomatic disorders and all bursts of negative emotions or self-limiting and self-sabotaging thoughts.

Internal emotional self-sabotage or black wolf arises when you focus on certain bursts of negative emotions or self-limiting thoughts that unbalance your energy system. This is where this emotional release technique comes into play and to begin the EFT - Tapping procedure the first thing we have to do is to prepare ourselves, recognize and measure the intensity of the problem.

*** Recognize the Problem:**

It can be given simply by thinking about it. In fact, to recognize means to reflect on it. Thinking about the problem and consciously focusing on it with a purpose in mind will bring up the altered states of consciousness that caused the knotted imbalances or disorders in your energy system.

Once we are aware of them, recognize the problem and accept it, then it is at that precise moment that these imbalances, disorders or stagnant energies can be unblocked. And to achieve that end is that we apply the basic recipe of EFT...

Recognizing the problem seems to be a very simple process. However, the reality is that you may find it a bit difficult to consciously think about it while tapping. It is for this reason that in applying this emotional release technique both preparation and measuring the intensity of the problem is an important part of the process. In the preparation to do the tapping, introducing a reminder phrase is fundamental, since this is the sentence or statement that we will repeat continuously while performing the basic or advanced EFT recipe...

*** The Reminder Phrase:**

It is simply a short sentence or statement that describes the problem to be solved. We repeat it out loud each time we tap on one of the vital points, meridians, or energetic channels of the basic or advanced EFT recipe sequence. In this way, we continually remind our system of the problem we are working on. The best reminder phrase we can usually use is the same one we chose as the sentence or statement for the affirmative part of the preparation phrase.

*** The Preparation Phrase:**

This is the stage where we gently rub the digit point located on the chest, called "the sensitive point", or we tap rhythmically on "the karate point" located on the instep of the hand. As we do this, we say loudly and clearly our preparation phrase three to seven times, as needed or as the occasion requires. For example: if you are working with fear of failure, the preparation statement would go something like this: "Even though I have this fear of failure, I love myself and accept myself completely and deeply just as I am.

*** EFT Tapping Sessions**:

They usually begin when we ourselves evaluate or measure the intensity of the problem on a scale from zero (0) to ten (10). Where zero (0) is equivalent to the highest possible state of well-being, while ten (10) would be equivalent to the maximum degree of intensity of the problem. This intensity measurement is always done before starting the tapping series and after applying the basic and advanced EFT recipe sequence. Whether it is a physical, mental, emotional, psychological, spiritual, or psychosomatic problem. One of the reasons why we evaluate or measure the intensity of the problem before starting the series and after applying the tapping sequence is to be able to determine how much progress is being made in each series or sequence of the emotional release technique.

*** Tips and Suggestions**:

The emotional release technique is very easy to use because it is a very flexible and adaptable procedure to multiple needs. For this reason, here I share with you some of the most important tips and suggestions to use EFT - Tapping effectively and thus amplify your experience and increase your chances of success with the practice of the technique.

- Be specific: the more specific you are, the better your experience will be and, therefore, the better the results will be. First, identify either the problem, the person, the place, the experience, the situation, the memories, the thoughts, the feelings, the emotions, or the specific sensation associated with the issue at hand and focus on it while performing the sequence or series of the preparatory affirmation.

- Measure the intensity of the problem: remember that it is important to assess the intensity of the problem you want to solve before you start. You can use an intensity meter on a scale from 0 to 10 (where zero (0) equals the highest possible state of well-being, while ten (10) would equal the maximum degree of intensity of the problem). To identify how strong your thoughts, feelings and emotions are around a specific problem, it is important to always do an intensity measurement before starting the tapping series and after applying the basic and advanced EFT recipe sequence. This action will allow you to measure your progress.

After you finish each round of EFT - Tapping, check your thoughts, feelings, and emotions again in relation to the previous state of intensity and evaluate whether they became stronger, or less strong, or stayed as they were. What is valuable with this procedure is that you should continue EFT Tapping until you achieve a zero (0) on this scale as an indicator of total release of the self-defeating limiting thoughts, feelings and emotions related to that particular issue.

- **Intensity testing**: after finishing a sequence of the basic EFT Tapping recipe, pay attention to any thoughts, feelings or emotions that come to your mind. It may be that a sensation of a part of the blockage appears, or you experience a memory about the issue you are releasing. If so, relax, relax, and run the basic EFT tapping sequence again until any thoughts, feelings or emotions are completely gone.

- **Be persistent**: repeat the basic and advanced EFT - Tapping recipe sequence until you completely release all limiting and self-defeating emotions associated with the specific problem. Occasionally there may be some aspects or layers of an energetic blockage or issue that still continue to manifest in some degree of intensity when the problem has been blocking our energetic channels for some time. For this reason, in these few cases, it is advisable to continue doing EFT - Tapping until all of them have been fully released.

- **Flexibility**: remember that you can do the rhythmic tapping on the EFT - Tapping points with either hand, either on the right or left side of your body, depending on how comfortable it is for you to practice the exercise.

- **The vital points or meridians**: if you tap rhythmically on the general area equivalent to the point, then you will activate and stimulate it. So, you can relax. If you have any doubts about the accuracy of the area you can relax and trust that EFT - Tapping will still work.

First Exercise:

1. **Preparation affirmation**: clearly specify the problem to be addressed in a short sentence while stimulating the karate point (Pk) or gently rubbing and massaging the sensitive point (Ps). Example: while pronouncing the preparation affirmation "Although I have this fear of failure, I love myself and

accept myself completely and deeply as I am", stimulate the karate point (Pk) or gently rub and massage the sensitive point (Ps).

2. **The negative sequence**: now put all your attention and focus on the problem to be addressed while stimulating the points of the basic EFT recipe sequence while at the same time repeating the reminder phrase out loud. This conscious action allows you to focus your mind on the problem, the limiting self-sabotaging emotion or negative thought pattern and thus allow tapping to release it.

Example of the reminder phrase: fear of failure: Start performing the sequence of the basic EFT recipe while at the same time tapping 3 to 7 times while repeating the reminder phrase "*Although I have this fear of failure, I love myself and accept myself completely and deeply as I am*". Below I share with you the abbreviations summarized for each vital point or meridian of the basic EFT recipe to be stimulated by tapping in the correct and corresponding order in which they are used.

Start by stimulating the crown point and follow the sequence of vital points or meridians to be stimulated through tapping.

- **Vital Points Crown "Co" and Face "Ce, Lo, Bo, Bn, Bl".**

Co = center of crown
TO = center of the forehead "**Third Eye**", "**Ajna** or **Sixth Chakra**".
Ce = beginning of eyebrow
Lo = side of the eye
Bo = under the eye
Bn = under the nose
Bl = under the lips

- **Vital Points Basic Recipe - Chest "Cl, Bb".**

Cl = clavicle = basic recipe
Bb = under the arm = basic recipe

- **The Advanced Vital Points Sore Spot or Pain Zone and Under the Chest or Under the Nipple (Ps - Zd) (Bp - Bt) and the Chakra** meridians: **Thymus - Heart, Above the Navel and Below the Navel (TC, MP, SV).**

Ps - Zd = tender point or painful area = advanced prescription.
TC = center of the chest "**Thymus-Heart**", "**Anahata or Fourth Chakra**".
Bp - Pt = under the breast "or" under the nipple = advanced prescription.

MP = above the navel "**Solar Plexus**", "**Manipura or Third Chakra**".
SV = below the navel "**Lower Abdomen**", "**Svadhisthana or Second Chakra**".

- **Vital Points Hand "Dp, Di, Dm or Dc, Me or Dme" - "Gm, Pk and Mñ or Mu" - "Gm, Pk and Mñ or Mu".**

Dp = thumb
Di = index finger
Dm or Dc = middle "or" middle finger
Me or Dme = little finger
Pg = range
Pk Pa= karate "o" friendship

- **Repeat the basic EFT recipe sequence - Tapping.**

Pk or Pa= karate point or friendship point
Ps or **Zd**= tender point or painful area
Mñ or **Mu** = Wrist Point.

3. **The positive sequence**: state and decree out loud the options, desired states, or alternative potential outcomes you wish to incorporate into your mental and psychological structure while stimulating through tapping on the points of the basic EFT recipe sequence to focus on the solution. This action allows you to incorporate a positive thought pattern and create a new, more empowered neural connection.

Example: *"I am on my way to success and personal excellence".* Tap the points in the EFT basic recipe sequence 3 to 7 times while repeating the positive reminder phrase *"I am on my way to success and personal excellence".*

Again, start by stimulating the crown point and follow the same sequence above of the vital points to be stimulated through tapping.

- **Vital Points Crown "Co" and Face "Ce, Lo, Bo, Bn, Bl".**

Co = center of crown
TO = center of the forehead "**Third Eye**", "**Ajna** or **Sixth Chakra**".
Ce = beginning of eyebrow
Lo = side of the eye
Bo = under the eye
Bn = under the nose
Bl = under the lips

- **Vital Points Basic Recipe - Chest "Cl, Bb".**

Cl = clavicle = basic recipe
Bb = under the arm = basic recipe

- **The Advanced Vital Points Sore Spot or Pain Zone and Under the Chest or Under the Nipple (Ps - Zd) (Bp - Bt) and the Chakra meridians: Thymus - Heart, Above the Navel and Below the Navel (TC, MP, SV).**

Ps - Zd = tender point or painful area = advanced prescription.
TC = center of the chest "**Thymus-Heart**", "**Anahata** or **Fourth Chakra**".
Bp - Pt = under the breast "or" under the nipple = advanced prescription.

MP = above the navel "**Solar Plexus**", "**Manipura** or **Third Chakra**".
SV = below the navel "**Lower Abdomen**", "**Svadhisthana** or **Second Chakra**".

- **Vital Points Hand "Dp, Di, Dm or Dc, Me or Dme" - "Gm, Pk and Mñ or Mu" - "Gm, Pk and Mñ or Mu".**

Dp = thumb
Di = index finger

Dm or Dc = middle "or" middle finger

Me or Dme = little finger

Pg = range

Pk Pa= karate "o" friendship

- **Repeat the basic EFT recipe sequence - Tapping.**

Pk or Pa= karate point or friendship point

Ps or **Zd**= tender point or painful area

Mñ or **Mu** = Wrist Point.

4. **Concentrate, focus on the exercise and connect with the positive reminder phrase**: *"I am on my way to success and personal excellence"*, breathe, inhale and exhale deeply while performing EFT - Tapping to facilitate the movement of energy throughout the body and balance the energetic channels.

Second Exercise:

Step 1: describe the specific problem, whether physical, mental, emotional, psychological, spiritual, or psychosomatic, for example: "headache", "phobia of spiders", "fear of heights" or "feelings of guilt, anger or sadness".

Step 2: assesses the level of intensity of the problem on a scale from 0 to 10 (where zero (0) equals the highest possible state of well-being, while ten (10) would be the maximum degree of intensity of the problem).

Step 3: repeat aloud three to seven times the following phrase which we will call "preparation phrase" replacing the blank space with the specific problem to work on, while at the same time stimulating the karate point (Pk) or gently rubbing and massaging the sensitive point (Ps). "Even though I have this _______________, I love myself and accept myself completely and deeply just as I am."

Examples:

"Even though I have this headache, I love myself and accept myself completely and deeply as I am."

"Even though I have this phobia of spiders, I love myself and accept myself completely and deeply just the way I am."

"Even though I have this fear of heights, I love myself and accept myself completely and deeply as I am."

"Even though I have this feeling of guilt, anger or sadness, I love myself and accept myself completely and deeply just as I am."

First Tapping Sequence:

Step 4: apply between 3, 5 or 7 gentle taps on each of the points of the following chart while repeating a phrase that summarizes the problem to be addressed, which for the purpose of the exercise we will call a "reminder phrase". Following the aforementioned examples above we could use the following: "headache", "phobia of spiders" and "fear of heights".

Repeat the basic EFT recipe sequence - Tapping:

- **Vital Points Crown "Co" and Face "Ce, Lo, Bo, Bn, Bl".**

Co = center of crown
TO = center of the forehead "**Third Eye**", "**Ajna** or **Sixth Chakra**".
Ce = beginning of eyebrow
Lo = side of the eye
Bo = under the eye
Bn = under the nose
Bl = under the lips

- **Vital Points Basic Recipe - Chest "Cl, Bb".**

Cl = clavicle = basic recipe
Bb = under the arm = basic recipe

- **The Advanced Vital Points Sore Spot or Pain Zone and Under the Chest or Under the Nipple (Ps - Zd) (Bp - Bt) and the Chakra meridians: Thymus - Heart, Above the Navel and Below the Navel (TC, MP, SV).**

Ps - Zd = tender point or painful area = advanced prescription.
TC = center of the chest "**Thymus-Heart**", "**Anahata** or **Fourth Chakra**".
Bp - Pt = under the breast "or" under the nipple = advanced prescription.

MP = above the navel "**Solar Plexus**", "**Manipura** or **Third Chakra**".

SV = below the navel "**Lower Abdomen**", "**Svadhisthana** or **Second Chakra**".

- **Vital Points Hand "Dp, Di, Dm or Dc, Me or Dme" - "Gm, Pk and Mñ or Mu" - "Gm, Pk and Mñ or Mu".**

Dp = thumb
Di = index finger
Dm or Dc = middle "or" middle finger
Me or Dme = little finger
Pg = range
Pk Pa= karate "o" friendship

- **Repeat the basic EFT recipe sequence - Tapping.**

Pk or **Pa**= karate point or friendship point
Ps or **Zd**= tender point or painful area
Mñ or **Mu** = Wrist Point.

The Procedure of the 4 Finger Points and the 9 Ranges:

Step 5: continuously stimulate the finger points (the energy or meridian points of the thumb, index, middle and little finger are located laterally in line with the base of the nail) and the gamma point *(point located just before the knuckles of the little and ring fingers in line with the central point between these two)* by gently tapping while keeping your head upright and performing the following actions:

1) close your eyes
2) open your eyes again
3) look down and to the right
4) look down and to the left
5) turn your eyes in a clockwise circle.
6) rotate the eyes in a counterclockwise circle.

7) hum a song for three seconds with your mouth closed.

8) count rapidly in ascending order from 1 to 5

9) hum a song again

10) count rapidly down from 5 to 1

Vital points of the fingers and gamma point of the hand:

Dp = thumb

Di = index finger

Dm or Dc = middle or middle finger

Me or Dme = little finger

Pg = range point

Second tapping sequence:

Step 6: reapply the basic EFT - Tapping recipe sequence as described in "step 4" while repeating the "reminder phrase".

Next rounds of tapping:

Step 7: check the changes that have occurred by re-evaluating the intensity of the problem on a scale from 0 to 10 (where zero (0) equals the highest possible state of well-being, while ten (10) would equal the maximum degree of intensity of the problem).

Subsequent applications of the treatment: if the intensity of the problem has decreased, but some thoughts, feelings and emotions still remain, it will be necessary to change the preparation sentence and the reminder sentence, adapting them to what remains of the original problem, adding the phrases still and the rest of "or" what remains following the following model.

Preparation phrase:

"Even though I still have this headache, I love and accept myself completely just the way I am" ...

"Even though I still have this phobia of spiders, I love and accept myself completely the way I am" ...

"Although I still have this fear of heights, I love and accept myself completely just the way I am" ...

"Even though I still have this feeling of guilt, anger or sadness, I love and accept myself completely just the way I am" ...

Reminder sentence:

"Although I still have the rest of this headache, I love and accept myself completely just the way I am" ...

"Although I still have what's left of this spider phobia, I love and accept myself completely just the way I am"...

"Although I still have the rest of this fear of heights, I love and accept myself completely just the way I am"...

"Even though I still have what's left of this feeling of guilt, anger or sadness, I love and accept myself completely as I am"...

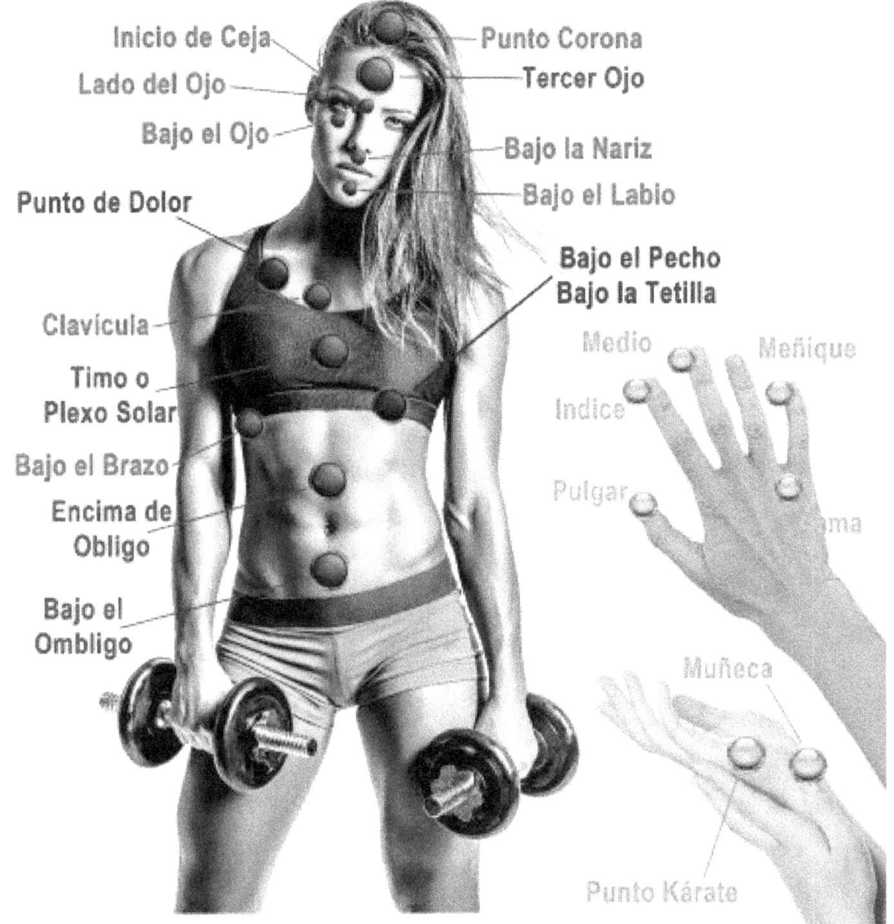

Basic Recipe, Advanced Stitches and Range Stitches: Image Appendix No. 1.

CHAPTER V: FINDING INNER PEACE: RELAXATION, MEDITATION AND MINDFULNESS TECHNIQUES

Part One: Inner Harmony: An Approach to Relaxation, Meditation and Mindfulness

Relaxation, meditation, and mindfulness are essential components of energetic and emotional healing methods, providing additional benefit for people who are stressed, busy and disconnected from their life purpose. What I like about these types of alternative therapies is that they do not require any sophisticated equipment, which makes them one of the most accessible methodologies for those who wish to master energetic-emotional healing, and achieve a balance between mind and body, thought and emotion.

Recent studies, conducted in prestigious universities, have established a relationship between heart disease, stress, anxiety, and factors such as anger, irritability, physical and mental exhaustion. As well as overwork and disconnection from our fundamental priorities to problems of energetic knots, stagnation of Chi or energetic flow and emotional problems, which finally materialize in manifest diseases.

For example, it has been shown that excessive stress can cause ischemia, which can lead to a heart attack and a host of other diseases, symptoms, and health disorders.

Therefore, relaxation, meditation and mindfulness take on additional importance in this context. Controlling anger, negative attitude, work stress, discouragement, anxiety, and overwork are essential for heart health and the overall well-being of the individual. As a result, developing the habit of relaxation, meditation and mindfulness can help you control and counteract these harmful effects. Below I will share some vital studies that demonstrate how applying relaxation, meditation and mindfulness techniques plays a role in the care of both physical and emotional health and well-being.

Over the years, numerous research studies have supported the benefits of meditation and relaxation for our health and well-being. These studies, conducted by some of the world's most prestigious universities, provide us with scientific insight into how these practices can transform our lives.

At Harvard University, for example, a 2011 study found that meditation can have a direct impact on our brains. Participants who completed an eight-week mindfulness-based stress reduction course showed an increase in gray matter density in the hippocampus, a part of the brain crucial for learning and memory. In addition, changes were observed in brain structures related to self-awareness, compassion, and introspection.

On the other hand, Johns Hopkins University conducted an analysis in 2014 that revealed that meditation can provide relief for anxiety and depression symptoms similar to that provided by antidepressants. This finding is especially relevant in a world where more and more people are seeking natural and effective alternatives to manage these disorders.

Since 1979, the University of Massachusetts Medical Center has been using mindfulness meditation in its Mindfulness-Based Stress Reduction Program. This program has helped countless patients deal with pain and a variety of health conditions, demonstrating the power of meditation in improving quality of life.

Finally, the University of California, Los Angeles (UCLA) School of Medicine has a Center for Research and Education in Relaxation, Breathing, Meditation and Mindfulness that has published numerous studies on the benefits of meditation and mindfulness in various populations. Their research has shown how these practices can benefit people with cancer, post-traumatic stress disorder and anxiety disorders.

These are just a few examples of the growing body of research that supports the benefits of meditation and relaxation for health and well-being. Through regular practice, we can harness these benefits to improve our own lives and achieve a state of inner peace and balance.

Part Two: The Art of Tranquility: Exploring Relaxation, Meditation, Mindfulness, and other alternatives.

One form of relaxation is transcendental meditation or mindfulness. Recent studies have shown that this method may reduce clogging of the arteries, a major cause of heart attack and stroke. People practice transcendental meditation or mindfulness by repeating soothing sounds while meditating, with the goal of achieving total relaxation. The researchers found that practitioners of transcendental meditation or mindfulness significantly reduced the thickness of their arterial wall compared to those who did not practice any relaxation technique.

Another study on progressive relaxation and mindful meditation seems to indicate that these techniques can reduce hypertension. These activities activate various bodily functions that allow the brain to release chemical compounds known as endorphins. Endorphins help relax muscles, relieve panic, decrease pain, and reduce anxiety.

Yoga, for example, is another relaxation method that requires mindfulness and can have similar effects to meditation. In one study, participants were subjected to several minutes of mental stress. They were then exposed to various relaxation techniques, such as listening to nature sounds or classical music, practicing yoga, progressive relaxation, and mindful meditation. Those who meditated mindfully, accompanying their meditation with breathing techniques, as well as those who practiced some yoga postures, significantly reduced the time it took for their blood pressure to return to normal. Thus, yoga, as a form of progressive relaxation and an act of mindfulness, is very effective.

On the other hand, breathing, meditation and mindfulness are simpler methods to achieve the same goal. Consequently, in this chapter we will focus on them. A study conducted at Stanford University showed that breathing and meditation influence almost every aspect of us, affecting our mind, our mood, and our body. By simply concentrating on your breathing while meditating, after some time you will be able to feel its effects immediately.

It is important to note that there are several breathing techniques and various methods of meditation. Each of these has been shown to help you reduce stress, fatigue, and anxiety.

Another simple way to relax is to exercise. If you are feeling irritable, a simple half hour of exercise will usually calm you down. Although exercise is an excellent way to lose weight, it does not teach proper stress management. Exercise should also be used in conjunction with another method of relaxation.

Receiving a massage is an unbeatable way to relax. To achieve full relaxation, it is necessary to surrender completely to the manipulation and touch of a professional therapist. There are several types of massages that provide different levels of relaxation. You just have to find the one you like the most.

Hypnosis is a very powerful relaxation technique. It is a good alternative for people who feel they have no idea how it feels to be relaxed. It is also a good option for people with health problems related to stress, anxiety, and others.

These relaxation techniques are just some of the ways to achieve relaxation. Another reason we need to relax, in addition to lowering blood pressure and reducing the chances of stroke and heart attack, is because stress produces hormones that suppress the immune system; relaxation gives the immune system time to recover and thus function more effectively.

Relaxation reduces the activity of the limbic system of the brain, which is the emotional center of our brain. In addition, the brain periodically needs more pronounced activity in the right hemisphere. Relaxation is one way to achieve this.

In short, relaxation can be really helpful once it is regularly incorporated into your lifestyle. Choose a technique that you feel you can practice regularly. And start transforming your life.

Part Three: The Power of Stillness: Relaxation, Meditation and Mindfulness Techniques

Meditation is a state in which the body and mind are consciously relaxed and focused. Practitioners of this art claim that it increases awareness, attention, and concentration, in addition to fostering a more positive attitude towards life.

Meditation is often associated with monks, mystics, and other spiritual disciplines. However, you don't need to be a monk or a mystic to enjoy its benefits, nor do you even need to be in a special place to practice it. You can even try it from the comfort of your own home.

Although there are many different approaches to meditation, the fundamental principles remain constant. The most relevant of these principles is to eliminate obstructive, negative, and wandering thoughts and fantasies, and to calm the mind with a deep sense of concentration and mindfulness. This purifies the mind of debris and prepares it for higher quality activity and emotional release.

Negative thoughts such as: those provoked by noisy neighbors, co-workers, bossy people, parking tickets or unwanted mail are considered to "pollute" the mind and leaving them aside allows it to "cleanse" itself so that it can focus on deeper, more meaningful thoughts. They contribute to "contaminate" the mind and leaving them aside allows to "clean" it so that it can focus on deeper and more meaningful thoughts.

At first it may seem deafening, and even impossible; since, we are all used to hearing and seeing things constantly, but as you develop the habit of relaxing, meditating, and concentrating on your breathing, you will find that you become more and more aware of everything around you.

If you find the meditation or yoga postures that you see on television intimidating, relax, they are not necessary to achieve the goal we want. Which is relaxation and full consciousness. The essential thing you should know is that the principle to perform a good meditation is to adopt a comfortable posture for you, which favors the concentration and stillness of your mind. You can sit with your legs crossed, you can stand while riding a public transportation unit, lying on your bed, or even walking.

What you should take into consideration is that the posture you adopt and the situation in which you do it, allows you to relax and concentrate, that would be a good starting point. Sitting or standing, in the comfort of your home, or in a bustling moment while on your way to work or school. You just have to feel comfortable, see the most conducive place for you, the most suitable posture that you feel comfortable with and the situation.

Loose and comfortable clothing helps a lot in the process. If you are just starting out, the place where you do the meditation should have a relaxing atmosphere. It can be the living room, bedroom, or any other place where you feel comfortable. And as you gain more experience, and awareness. You will see how you will be able to meditate, while doing another activity. This is a more advanced level, of course, but it is possible. Maintaining stillness and inner peace, even in the hustle and bustle of everyday life, will help you maintain your psycho-emotional balance.

To start developing the habit of relaxation, meditation, and mindfulness, you may want to arrange the room in a way that is soothing to your senses. Silence helps most people to relax and meditate, so it is advisable to have a quiet, secluded area away from the ringing of the telephone or the hum of the washing machine. Pleasant smells can also help in this regard, so having scented candles on hand is an excellent idea.

The monks seen on television emitting these monotonous sounds are actually reciting their mantra. This, in simple terms, is a simple sound that, for these practitioners, has a mystical value. However, in everyday life, these practices are not necessary to perform; however, it is worth noting that focusing on repeated actions, such as breathing and humming a mantra, helps the practitioner to enter a higher state of consciousness.

The principle is concentration. In your particular case, you can try to concentrate on a particular object or thought, or even, keeping your eyes open, concentrate on your breathing.

An example of a routine would be, in a meditative state, to silently name each part of your body and concentrate your awareness on it. As you do this, you should be aware of any tension in any part of your body. Mentally visualize the release of that tension. And you will see, with time and practice, it works wonders.

In short, meditation is a relatively risk-free practice, and its benefits are well worth giving it a try. Studies have shown that relaxation, conscious breathing, meditation, and mindfulness have beneficial physiological effects on the body. And there has been a growing consensus in the medical community to continue studying its positive health effects.

Part Four: The Path to Serenity: A Journey through Relaxation, Meditation and Mindfulness Techniques.

To continue with this fascinating topic and move on to practice. I will share with you "5 Relaxation, Breathing, Meditation and Mindfulness Techniques to Reduce Stress".

*** 5 Relaxation, Breathing, Meditation and Mindfulness Techniques to Reduce Stress.**

Relaxation, Breathing, Meditation and Mindfulness techniques have gained notoriety in recent years because they are part of a psychological process in which people are able to focus their mind and, thus, improve their personal, academic, professional or any other area.

For this reason, large international companies have implemented, for some time now, Relaxation, Breathing, Meditation and Mindfulness methods to reduce stress, as well as to improve the performance of their employees and their well-being.

Here are nine simple basic techniques of Relaxation, Breathing, Meditation and Mindfulness to reduce stress, which can also help you optimize your time and improve your performance in any activity:

1. Immerse Hands in Warm Water.

According to Charlie Knoles, a specialist in meditation and Relaxation, Breathing, Meditation and Mindfulness, rubbing the hands strongly in warm water is a practice that generates calmness in the person. This will help to open the blood vessels and, with this, eliminate the state of stress in the brain. Unblocking the energetic knots and making your vital energy flow, revitalizing your mind and thoughts.

2. Breathe Slowly, Consciously, and attentively.

Although it sounds very obvious, it is an important practice. When people are stressed, they tend to take short, sharp breaths automatically, but that's not necessarily beneficial to your well-being. Our nervous systems are wired in such a way that: inhalation is linked to the stress response and exhalation to the relaxation response, Knoles explains. So, taking a short inhale and emphasizing a long exhale consciously helps, prevents classic stress responses, such as adrenaline or insomnia, from kicking in. And in turn, by being conscious of the act of breathing, we activate our parasympathetic, and as a result, we improve the secretion of hormones such as serotonin or noradrenaline, which are beneficial for the body and for general well-being.

3. Observe an Object and Concentrate (Focus on a Point).

Choose an object (if it is natural, all the better) from your immediate environment and concentrate on looking at it for a minute or two. This could be a flower, an insect, or even the clouds or the moon. Focus, direct your attention to that object you are observing to relax and concentrate (focus) on this activity. You can analyze each characteristic of that object, which will help exercise your mind to learn to concentrate on one thing at a time. And this, my dear ones, is what we call mindfulness, being in the HERE and the NOW.

4. Listening to Music. Binaural waves.

Listening to music can modify repetitive thought patterns. "It can be classical music, ambient music, or nature sounds, or soft music, which you like, inspires and relaxes you." The important thing is to avoid loud sounds, and any rhythms that may trigger stress responses. Listening to music can serve as a method you can use at home or work, as long as your office allows you to listen to music for some period of time. On the other hand, there are binaural sounds, which have been shown to have a positive effect on the brain, stimulating the hemispheres and activating areas of the brain that are beneficial to health. Among the best-known binaural odes, we have: Alpha frequencies, 8 hertz, key to brain activity, bringing numerous benefits such as increased creativity, improved memory, increased concentration, and greater relaxation. Stimulating certain types of brainwaves can have positive effects in specific areas of daily life. For example, better sleep quality is associated with delta waves. Theta waves are related to emotional healing and personal empowerment. Gamma and beta waves relate to better academic and work performance. Ideally, use the frequency that suits your needs at any given time, you can try each frequency in different situations.

5. Eat a Snack Slowly (enjoy the present moment).

Another simple exercise you can do in everyday places is this. Slowly eat a small snack, perceive, and enjoy that chocolate or fruit. Use all your senses to see it, touch it, smell it, and feel it. Savor its texture, its flavor, how it feels in your mouth. After ingesting it, let your lips lift slightly and smile. The important thing is to connect with the here and now, in each bite, and enjoy the moment.

Exercises such as the above are just a few small examples of techniques related to mindfulness. This discipline, introduced in the West since the 1970s, has an increasing presence in academic articles, medical studies, and scientific research, but also in business management.

In today's urban environments, where work and personal pressures are very complex, the methods of Relaxation, Breathing, Meditation and Mindfulness become relevant to contribute to a valid alternative to counteract one of the major problems of today's societies: stress.

Here are three simple exercises that you can also incorporate into your daily routine.

6. Breathing Exercise:

1. Find a quiet, comfortable place to sit or lie down. Close your eyes if you feel comfortable doing so.

2. Begin to notice your breathing as it is, without trying to change it.

3. Now, slowly begin to make your inhalations and exhalations longer and deeper. Inhaling through your nose and exhaling through your mouth.

4. Try to make your inhales and exhales the same length. You can count to 4 as you inhale and then count to 4 as you exhale to help you do this.

5. Continue breathing in this way for a few minutes, keeping your attention on the flow of your breath.

6. If your mind starts to wander, simply bring it back to your breath.

7. Progressive Relaxation Exercise:

1. Find a quiet, comfortable place to sit or lie down. Close your eyes if you feel comfortable doing so.

2. Start by focusing on your feet. Tense the muscles in your feet for a few seconds and then relax them.

3. Next, move on to your calves. Tense and relax these muscles in the same way.

4. Continue this process with each muscle group in your body. Work from your feet to your legs, your torso, your arms, and finally your face.

5. As you relax each muscle group, you should begin to feel a sense of relaxation and calmness spreading throughout your body.

8. Guided Meditation Exercise:

1. Find a quiet, comfortable place to sit. Close your eyes if you are comfortable doing so.

2. Begin to concentrate on your breathing. Don't try to change it, just observe it as it is.

3. Now, imagine that you are in a place that you find very relaxing. It could be a beach, a forest, or even a favorite spot from your childhood.

4. Try to imagine this place as vividly as possible. What do you see? What do you hear? What smells are there?

5. If your mind starts to wander, gently bring it back to this site. Remember, there is no right or wrong way to do this. It is your personal space to relax.

6. You can stay in this spot for as long as you like. When you are ready to leave, take a few deep breaths and then slowly open your eyes.

I hope these exercises will be useful for your daily routines. Remember, the key to all these practices is patience and consistency. It's okay if you find it hard to concentrate at first. I assure you that, with time, it will get easier. Remember, repetition and practice are the key to success in developing good habits.

9. *Exercise of Self-Hypnosis or Guided Meditation.*

Start by finding a quiet, comfortable spot to sit or lie down. Make sure you will not be interrupted for the next few minutes.

Close your eyes and begin to concentrate on your breathing. Do not try to change it, just observe it as it is. Feel how the air enters and leaves your body, filling you with calm and tranquility.

Now, I want you to imagine a warm, bright light just above your head. This light represents peace and relaxation. Feel this light begin to pour over you, touching your skin and giving you a sense of calm and comfort.

The light begins to move downward, from the top of your head to the tips of your toes. As the light moves, you feel every part of your body relax and let go.

Feel the light pass across your forehead, relaxing all the muscles in your face. Your jaw loosens, your eyes relax.

The light moves down towards your neck and shoulders. Feel any tension in this area simply melt away.

The light continues to move down through your arms and into your hands. Feel your arms become heavy and relaxed.

The light moves to your chest and stomach. Feel how your breathing becomes deeper, and slower, more and more relaxed.

The light moves down through your legs and down to your feet. Feel your legs become heavy and relaxed.

Now, your whole body is bathed in this warm, soothing light. You feel completely calm and relaxed, completely at peace.

In this state of deep relaxation, your mind is open and receptive. Now it is time to repeat your affirmation or intention. It could be something like "I am at peace with myself and the world" or "Every day I feel more relaxed and calmer". Repeat this affirmation in your mind several times.

Now, I want you to imagine that you are in a very relaxing place. It could be a beach, a garden, or any place that makes you feel at peace. Spend some time in this place, enjoying the feeling of relaxation and peace it gives you.

When you are ready to come out of this state of self-hypnosis, begin to slowly wiggle your fingers and toes. Then, gently stretch your body and open your eyes. You will feel awake, refreshed and completely relaxed.

I hope this guided self-hypnosis session will be useful for your daily routine. Remember, self-hypnosis is a skill that develops with practice. The more you practice, the easier it will be for you to enter this state of deep relaxation.

FINAL WORDS

Congratulations, champions! We have reached the end of this wonderful book, a special edition that I have written with dedication for you. We have traveled together a long road of training and learning, a journey towards your success and personal fulfillment.

This book was created and designed, with you in mind, as a practical step-by-step instruction manual. It is intended to guide you through a mental process of continuous learning and training, using a well prepared and simplified "pattern of action". This pattern is designed to bring you optimal, effective, and permanent results through the tools and methodologies of energy healing.

I hope to see you in the next books of the series: "Universal Principles and Laws of Success". If this book, **"Inner Healing: Break Chains and Free Yourself from Inner Self Sabotage. *Learn to Strengthen Your Inner Warrior and Master Your Emotions and Thoughts*"**, has pleased you and you wish to share it, your help will allow us to reach more people. Thank you for your contribution.

Now is the time to start living a wonderful, principled life. Remember: take action and make things happen. And I promise you: Soon, you and I will find ourselves on the cusp of excellence.

Your great friend, **Ylich Tarazona**, wishes you well.

EPILOGUE AND INSPIRATIONAL WORDS

We have reached the end of this journey, but in reality, this is only the beginning. The path to inner healing and freedom from self-sabotage is a journey that continues throughout our lives. Each day presents us with new opportunities to learn, grow and heal.

This book has been a guide, a map that has shown you the way. But the real journey happens within you. It is you who must take the steps, face your fears, break your chains, and free yourself from self-sabotage. It is you who must strengthen your inner warrior and master your emotions and thoughts.

Remember, you are not alone on this journey. As the author of this book, I am with you in spirit, supporting you every step of the way. And don't forget, you always have the power to help yourself. You have the power to heal, to change, to grow. You have the power to be the best version of yourself.

So, as you close this book, I urge you not to close your mind and heart to the possibilities that await you. Keep hope, keep faith in yourself and keep moving forward. No matter what life throws at you, you always have the ability to overcome.

And remember, this is not the end. It is just the beginning of your new life, a life of healing, growth, and liberation. A life in which you are free to be yourself, free from self-sabotage, and free to reach your full potential.

I wish you all the best on your journey. May you find the healing, peace, and happiness you seek. And may you always remember that you have the power to heal yourself. With love and gratitude, **YLICH TARAZONA.**

ABOUT THE AUTHOR

Professional Background: YLICH TARAZONA is a renowned psychologist, hypnotherapist, writer, and international lecturer. He is also a Master Coach with NLP and Master Trainer in Neurolinguistic Programming. Specialized in alternative therapies, Ericksonian hypnosis, Emotional Freedom Technique (EFT - Tapping) and energy healing. He is considered one of the most prominent and influential professionals in the field of personal excellence by the various media.

He is destined to leave a legacy in the lives of millions of people through his passion, enthusiasm, dynamism, and principled leadership. He is the creator of Hypno Reengineering and Mental Bio Reprogramming, two online systems dedicated to providing coaching in the consolidation of competencies and development of maximum human potential.

Its methodology is designed to enhance the competencies of the individual through a sequence of sessions and therapies, which aim to guide the coachees to find the necessary tools that will allow them to reach their goals, achieve their objectives and consolidate results in their areas of excellence.

He is the author of the **Reengineering and Mental Bioprogramming** series of books and conferences, including: **"Program your mind and determine your future"**, **"Heal myself and free yourself from self-sabotage"**, **"The power of change and personal reinvention"**, **"Discover your purpose and find your destiny"**, **"The power of goals and the achievement of objectives"** and **"Consolidate your personal brand"**, among others.

He is also the creator of the book **"The Power of Hypnosis"** and the course **"Practical Hypnosis"**. These works deal with ancient and modern hypnosis in a professional, clear, and easy to understand way. His focus is on helping readers or participants understand what trance and hypnotic phenomena are, as well as sharing a wide variety of techniques, suggestions, inductions, suggestibility tests, covert tests, convincers and deepeners, therapeutic and linguistic elements used by the hypnotist or hypnotherapist to generate hypnotic states and bring about the necessary changes in the individual's subconscious mind.

In terms of his **PURPOSE**, **mission** and personal **vision**, YLICH TARAZONA aims to share with his readers the resources they need to move forward with determination, teaching them to clarify their ideas, set goals and develop action plans that will enable them to conquer their most cherished dreams, allowing them to create their own future, write the story of their own lives and forge their own destiny every step of the way.

His **MISSION** is to leave a mark that makes a difference in the lives of the people to whom he teaches and carries his message, transmitting a legacy that allows them to evolve in all the transcendental aspects of life, personally, spiritually, emotionally, professionally, academically, and financially.

His **VISION** is to bring people hope and a therapeutic option that allows them to transform their lives and improve, helping them to develop that seed of greatness that everyone carries inside, motivating them to develop their full human potential, to the next level of success, generating an improved version of themselves and opening new opportunities that allow them to rediscover themselves on the road to personal transformation.

"I firmly believe that within each of us lies a seed of greatness and a vast reservoir of unlimited potential that usually lies dormant, waiting to be discovered and developed, to blossom into our outer world. When each of us awakens that individual potential, we will rediscover our mission and the purpose that gives meaning to our lives, in a new conscious awakening. This is what I call, Reinvention and Personal Reengineering" **YLICH TARAZONA.**

Other Publications, Special Editions and Books Created by the Author

Dear reader, it was a pleasure to have shared with you this time of reading, I hope you have enjoyed to the maximum the information contained in this book that with so much affection I have prepared for you. Your great friend YLICH TARAZONA.

If you liked the content of my books and would like to know more about my other publications, here is a list of all my books.

Updated Book List (JULY 2023):

1. **"Awaken Your Greatness**: How to Program Your Mind to Discover Your Authentic Self". *Learn how to Transform your Life and Awaken your Inner Power.*

2. **"Inner Healing**: Break Chains and Free Yourself from Inner Self Sabotage". *Learn how to Strengthen your Inner Warrior and Master your Emotions and Thoughts.*

3. **"Reinvent Yourself**: The Magic of Personal Transformation". *Innovation and Empowerment of the Self to create an Improved Version of Yourself.*

4. **"Purpose and Destiny**: The Compass of your Existence". *Discover the Principles and Connections for Living a Purposeful Life.*

5. **"Make the Difference**: Position your Personal Brand at the Top". *Strategies to Stand Out in a Competitive World.*

6. **"Goals and Objectives**: The Art of Strategic Planning". *A Step-by-Step Guide to Consolidate Your Dreams and Achieve Success.*

7. **"Mental Re-Engineering**: The Art of Redesigning your Thoughts". *Learn how to Reprogram your Mind for Success and Begin your Personal Reinvention Process.*

8. **"Habits of Excellence**: The Path to Wholeness". *Secrets for a Healthy, Full and Happy Life.*

9. **"Inner Harmony**: Secrets of Life Coaching for a Life of Fulfillment and Balance." *From Self-Awareness to Success. A Step-by-Step Guide to Personal Growth.*

10. **"Transform Your Life with NLP**: A Practical Guide to Neurolinguistic Programming for Effective Personal Change." *Master Effective Techniques and Methodologies for Deep Personal Transformation.*

11. **"The Art of Persuasion**: Discover the Power of Figurative Language and Metaphors in Communication." *Become a Persuasive Communicator through the Power of Metaphors and Allegories.*

12. **"Applied Hypnosis**: A Practical Manual for Developing Hypnotic and Persuasive Skills." *Acquire the Skills to Hypnotize and Persuade Effectively and Ethically.*

13. **"Hypnotize Effectively**: A Practical Course for Mastering Hypnosis in Any Context." *Learn the Secrets to Hypnotize Anyone, Anytime, anywhere.*

14. **"Quantum Awakening**: Mental Reengineering and Bio-Programming for Personal Evolution and the New Age of Thought."

Make a Quantum Leap in your Personal Evolution and Open the Doors to the New Age of Thought.

15. "**Neuro-Oratory and Hypnotic Persuasion**: Discover the Art of Influencing with the Power of your Words." *Develop Persuasive Communication Skills and Power your Influence in Everyday Conversations.*

16. "**Engrams and Neural Consciousness**: Exploring the Relationship between the Conscious and Subconscious Mind." *Deepens the Relationship between Consciousness and Perception.*

17. "**The Power of the Subconscious Mind**: Take Control of your Thoughts and Program your Mind for Success." *Discover the Unlimited Potential of your Subconscious to Transform your Life.*

18. "**Master in Life Coaching with NLP**: Mastering Techniques and Methodologies for Goal Achievement." *Learn the Essential Coaching Tools to Guide Others to Success.*

19. "**Multilevel Network Marketing**: Discover Network Marketing Opportunities in the Digital Age" *Open your Path to Financial Freedom with Effective Network Marketing Strategies.*

Always keep in mind that: "Constant learning, continuous training and permanent study are the keys between those who achieve success and those who do not". **YLICH TARAZONA**.

You can contact me directly through my website:

https://ylichtarazona.org.es/

COPYRIGHTS

Don't miss out!

Visit the website below and you can sign up to receive emails whenever Ylich Tarazona publishes a new book. There's no charge and no obligation.

https://books2read.com/r/B-A-PAIU-ZPGLC

BOOKS 2 READ

Connecting independent readers to independent writers.

Did you love *Inner Healing*? Then you should read *Awaken Your Greatness*[1] by Ylich Tarazona!

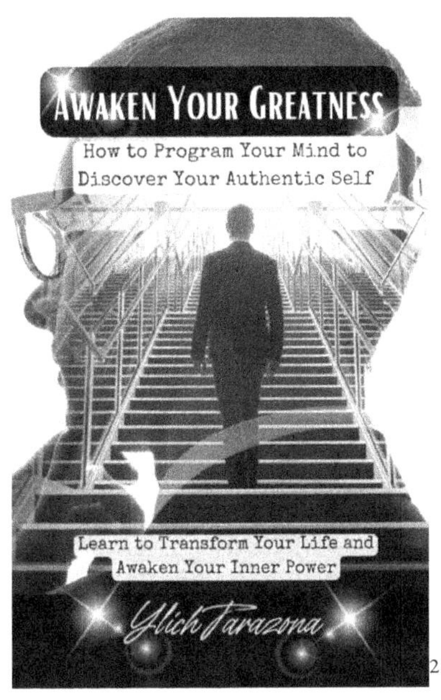

The Secret to Unleashing Your Potential and Determining Your Destiny!Are you ready to unleash your unlimited potential and conquer your boldest dreams? Let me introduce you to "Awaken Your Greatness: How to Program Your Mind to Discover Your Authentic Self," the ultimate personal development program that will take you from where you are now to where you have always desired to be.Imagine waking up every morning filled with energy, confidence, and determination to face any challenge that comes your way. With "Awaken Your Greatness: How to Program Your Mind to Discover Your Authentic Self," you will discover the most powerful and effective tools and strategies to transform your thoughts, emotions, and actions into unstoppable engines of success.This program is based on decades of research, as well as psychotherapeutic tools accompanied by extensive expertise and experience in the field of personal development, self-empowerment, self-help,

---

1. https://books2read.com/u/meXOer

2. https://books2read.com/u/meXOer

and achievement motivation. This book is designed to help you overcome your fears, overcome your limitations, and become the best version of yourself.Here, you will find more than mere theories; you will discover a set of practical techniques and methodologies backed by science and proven in real life. Additionally, you will learn how to reprogram your conscious and subconscious mind to eliminate limiting beliefs and adopt new, empowered thought patterns that propel you towards your success and personal fulfillment.And that's not all. "Awaken Your Greatness: How to Program Your Mind to Discover Your Authentic Self" will also provide you with a detailed action plan so you can implement what you have learned into your daily life. With interactive exercises, creative visualizations, and positive affirmations, you will strengthen your mental and emotional muscles in this process of self-discovery.Imagine the impact you will have on your career, personal relationships, and overall well-being when you become the master of your own destiny, the author of your own story, and the captain of your fate. You will no longer be a passive spectator in your life; you will become the protagonist of an epic tale that transcends time.Start taking control of your life. Act now and discover the power within you. Remember, you only have one life to live, and only you have the power to make it extraordinary. This is your moment to shine, to transcend your own limitations, and reach levels of success you never thought possible before.This journey of rediscovery will help you:

- Understand the different stages that give rise to the formation and development of self-esteem.

- Develop a healthy self-image and elevate your positive perception of yourself.

- Decipher and overcome limiting paradigms and self-destructive habits, creating new empowered mental maps.

- Reprogram your thoughts and your conscious and unconscious mental structure to align them with your dreams and goals of success.

- Reconfigure your beliefs, experiences, and competencies to enhance your innate abilities.

- Establish new patterns and habits of behavior that will propel you toward a higher level of consciousness.

- Take action, manifest your reality, and start living an extraordinary life based on principles.

- NLP Techniques o neurolinguistic programming.

It's time to awaken your inner power, learn to attract what you deserve in your life, and become the architect of your own reality. So, get ready to transform your life! Your greatness awaits, so act now and awaken your inner greatness!

Read more at https://ylichtarazona.com.es/.

Also by Ylich Tarazona

Chronicles of the Guardians: In Search of the Sacred Relics
Chronicles of the Guardians: In Search of the Sacred Relics

CRÓNICAS DE LOS GUARDIANES: En Búsqueda de las Reliquias Sagradas
Crónicas de los Guardianes: En Búsqueda de las Reliquias Sagradas

Maestría en Oratoria y Comunicación Persuasiva
El Poder de Persuadir con tus Palabras

Principes de base du succès et lois préliminaires du succès
Reprogrammez votre esprit et déterminez votre destin

Principi di base per il successo e leggi preliminari del successo
Riprogramma la tua mente e determina il tuo destino

Princípios Básicos para o Sucesso e Leis Preliminares do Sucesso

Reprograme a sua mente e determine o seu destino

Principios Básicos para Triunfar y Leyes Preliminares del Éxito
¡Guía de Autoayuda y Superación Personal!

Principios Psicoterapéuticos para Triunfar y ser Feliz
Hijos Triunfadores - Guía Psicoterapéutica para Padres

Principios y Leyes Universales del Éxito
Despierta Tu Grandeza
Sanación Interior

Principles and Universal Laws of Success
Awaken Your Greatness
Inner Healing

Psychotherapeutic Principles for Success and Happiness
Successful Sons Psychotherapeutic Guide for Parents
Self-help and Self-Improvement Guide!

Reengineering and Mental Reprogramming
Personal Reinvention
Reprogram Your Mind and Determine Your Destiny
The Power to Heal Yourself
Discover Your Life Purpose

The Power of Goals
How to Build Your Personal Brand

Reingeniería y Reprogramación Mental
Reinvención Personal. El Arte de Rediseñar tú Vida
El Poder de Sanarte a Ti Mismo
Descubre Tu Propósito de Vida
El Poder De Las Metas
Cómo Construir Tu Marca Personal
Reprograma Tu Mente y Determina Tu Destino

Standalone
Despierta Tus Capacidades Oníricas
Awaken Your Dreaming Capabilities
Hábitos de Excelencia Para Vivir Una Vida Saludable
Habits of Excellence for Living a Healthy Life

Watch for more at https://ylichtarazona.com.es/.

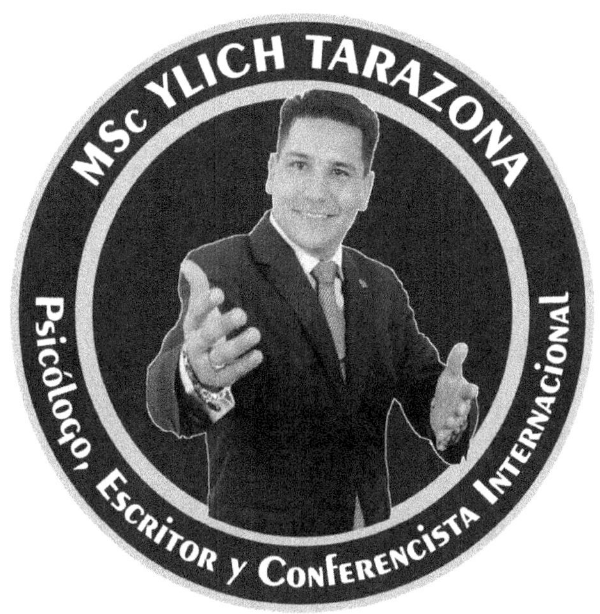

About the Author

YLICH TARAZONA reconocido, Psicólogo, Hipnoterapeuta Gestalt, Conferencista Internacional y Escritor, Autor de la Serie Reingeniería y Reprogramación Mental.

Máster Coach con PNL y Trainer en PROGRAMACIÓN NEUROLINGÜÍSTICA. Especialista en Terapias Alternativas. Hipnosis Ericksoniana, Técnica de Liberación Emocional (EFT - Tapping), Sanación Energética, Biodescodificación y Medicina Germánica.

Considerado en los distintos medios de comunicación como uno de los profesionales más destacado e influyente dentro del campo de la EXCELENCIA PERSONAL. Destinado a ejercer un legado en la vida de cientos de personas a través de su PASIÓN, ENTUSIASMO, DINAMISMO y LIDERAZGO centrado en principios.

C.E.O. Fundador de HIPNO REINGENIERÍA y BIO REPROGRAMACIÓN MENTAL ® Un Salto Cuántica para la Evolución del SER y el Despertar de la Consciencia.

Uno de los SISTEMAS ONLINE dedicado a brindar COACHING en la CONSOLIDACIÓN de Competencias y Desarrollo del Máximo Potencial Humano. Especializados en el Entrenamiento, Formación y Adiestramiento de alto nivel a través de las técnicas de la Hipnosis Ericksoniana, la Programación Neurolingüística y la Reingeniería Mental.

Nuestra metodología está diseñada para potenciar las competencias del individuo por medio de una secuencia de sesiones y terapias. Que tienen como objetivo guiar a los coachee a encontrar las herramientas necesarias que les permitan Alcanzar sus Metas. Concretar sus Objetivos y Consolidar Resultados Eficaces de Óptimo Desempeño en un campo de acción específico (Áreas de Excelencia).

Con el objetivo de obtener logros significativos de manera más efectiva, acompañamos nuestro proceso de HIPNO REINGENIERÍA y BIO REPROGRAMACIÓN MENTAL ® con Sesiones de Life Coaching. Técnicas de PNL o Programación Neurolingüística, Reingeniería Mental, Hipnoterapia Ericksoniana, Técnicas de Liberación Emocional y Sanación Energética Cuántica adaptadas para tal fin.

Read more at https://ylichtarazona.com.es/.

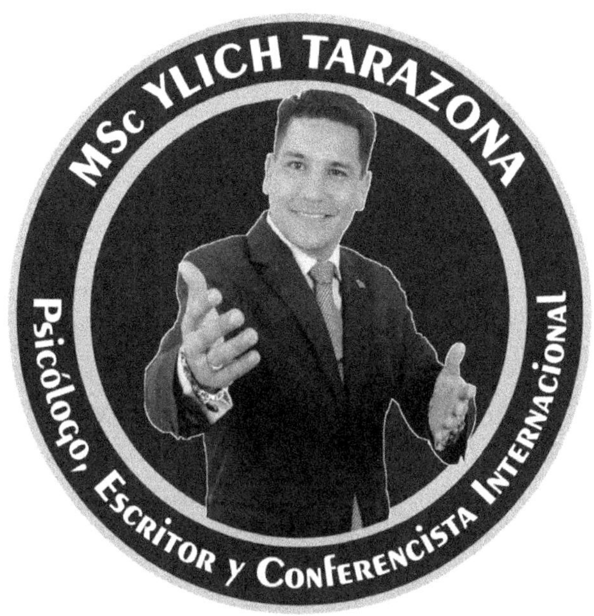

About the Publisher

Hola, permíteme presentarme. Soy **Ylich Tarazona**, un psicólogo, hipnoterapeuta, conferencista internacional y escritor. Mi pasión por el desarrollo humano me ha llevado a crear obras significativas como la serie **«Principios Básicos para Triunfar y Leyes Preliminares del Éxito»** que se componen de 7 libros extraordinarios que están enfocados en el empoderamiento del ser.

Además de mis estudios como psicólogo, me especialicé como **Máster Coach con PNL** y **Trainer en Programación Neurolingüística**. También tuve la oportunidad de especializarme en terapias alternativas, como: **Hipnosis ericksoniana**, técnica de liberación emocional (EFT-Tapping) y **sanación energética**. Lo que me permite poder emplear una variedad de metodologías, haciendo más efectivas mis aportaciones.

Se me ha reconocido en varios medios de comunicación como una de las figuras más destacadas en el campo de la excelencia personal. Gracias a mi pasión, entusiasmo, dinamismo y liderazgo centrado en principios. **Valores que están orientados a generar un impacto duradero en la vida de innumerables personas.**

Así mismo, soy el creador de un innovador sistema de Reingeniería y Bioprogramación Mental ®, un salto cuántico para la evolución del ser y el despertar de la conciencia.

Mi sistema de **Reingeniería y Bioprogramación Mental** ® es una metodología diseñada para ayudar a las personas a consolidar habilidades esenciales y desarrollar el máximo de su potencial humano. Gracias a que empleamos estratégicamente una serie de herramientas de **life coaching** combinadas con técnicas avanzadas de **hipnosis ericksoniana** y **programación neurolingüística**. Permite a los participantes obtener los resultados deseados.

Nuestra metodología única está diseñada para fortalecer las habilidades individuales de cada persona a través de una serie de sesiones y terapias. **El objetivo de este proceso de acompañamiento es guiar a cada cliente individualmente a encontrar las herramientas necesarias para alcanzar sus metas, materializar sus objetivos y obtener resultados efectivos en sus áreas de excelencia.**